Pinnacle Of Life

Kishore Shanbhag

First Edition

Copyright © Kishore Shanbhag 2020

All rights reserved.

ISBN: 9798633084597

Dedicated to my little family.

CONTENTS

	Personal Notes	3
1	The Great Certainty.	9
2	A Bucket List.	27
3	It is Your Choice.	47
4	Influence of Religion.	67
5	Memento mori.	87
6	Long life and Immortality.	105
7	Culture Customs and Belief.	121
8	Care and Cure.	137
9	What happens when I die?	155
10	Facing Bereavement.	173
11	Solving the Final Mystery.	191
	Epilogue – Pillars of Wisdom	207
	Inspiration	215

Pinnacle of Life

List of Poems

1.	I Bow Thee.	7
2.	Looking at Death.	25
3.	Into Emptiness.	45
4.	COVID on my Ward.	65
5.	Elements.	85
6.	Platonic Love.	104
7.	Dualism.	120
8.	Care Home.	136
9.	No Surprise.	**1**54
10.	Me and My Soul.	171
11.	Know How.	190
12.	Wisdom.	206

PINNACLE

OF

LIFE

PERSONAL NOTES

Introduction

There is an acute need to reinvent death. For too long, humans have suffered from anxiety and fear around end of life. The grief and sense of loss suffered by the near and dear people around a dying person have been exploited by super powers, religions, hierarchical structures, medical science and intellectuals. Uncertainty around the process of dying forced leaders and thinkers, for centuries, to come up with some explanation about the natural phenomenon. Unfortunately, the solutions proposed further added to the negative thinking, fear and darkness around the process of death. Creation of concepts of hell, sin, torture, punishment and painful death further reinforced the anxiety.

END OF LIFE also created immediate sense of loss of control, anger, frustration and grief. Perhaps there was a need for the society to pretend to have some control over the events of death. To dissipate the anger and give some space for the grieving, that the loss was gradual and not sudden, a notion was created that the death was not the end. This led to creation of an entity termed soul, atman or spirit which would leave the body of the diseased, but would linger around, depending on what scripture you subscribed to. Some believed your spirit, after death would reunite with a super spirit, others created a special place like heaven for it to reside. Also, the concept of recycling the spirit either as reincarnation or cyclical events of rebirths were invented. These reassured humans that death was not an end, but merely a stage of life cycle.

There is a need to talk about the truth. Talk about dying. As it actually happens. As it actually affects the dying, and the people around. Removing the deep entrenched beliefs, cultural and religious, unwrapping the mystic and supernatural, we need to discuss death as a natural phenomenon. I hope this will help in alleviating the anxiety and lift the darkness around the dying. It will help people to lead a better life, greener, humane and happy, not worrying about impending doom of hell and horror. The need to remove the false hope of angels and virgins, and to replace it with a true hope, a hope of peace and with recognition of truth, is urgent. Religion gives solace and framework to the society, we have to absorb those great qualities, at the same time free people of superstitious beliefs and anxiety.

NATURE always chooses when you die. But understanding of biology, medicine and even human thought process, combined with technology and social media has changed the way humans lived since birth of civilisation. We control everything in life, when we are born, how we look, whom we share our thoughts with, and even where our nutrition comes from. We have degree of choice on everything we do in life, why not have the same degree of control and choice over the most important event of your life. With some radical thinking, both individual level and talking about it to the family and friends, you can achieve true nirvana, the liberation from the anxiety of death.

Beware of another important fact. In spite of all the advances in medicine, we can't cure all ailments, can't nurse all pain and avoid the inevitable. In fact, modern medicine is capable of inflicting torturous damage in pursuit of isolated success. It is easy to lose the bigger picture, person's best interest. Patients, families and doctors alike need to understand when to let go. Sometimes that is the most difficult decision to make for everyone concerned. *Medicalisation of death has done more harm than the spiritualisation of it.*

In the final chapter, I have attempted to give an example of small steps you can take to become more aware and prepared, so that the end of life, whenever it comes, it will not be a shock. Of course, everyone has their own way, you know what is your personal life path, the book only makes you to think about one. As a society, there is a need for us to change our attitude towards death and dying. Need to put in place support, help people to plan their demise. Planned, pain free, peaceful end of life is in every human being's interest. Death is such a significant event of life that we can't allow unseen, unknown powers to take control of it. My book is an attempt to empower people to take control towards their final journey, death, the pinnacle of life.

An apology

I appreciate that the text and thoughts expressed in this book are not to the liking of everyone. The text is written largely atheistic or agnostic tone and I would like to acknowledge the fact that many of you may wish to follow more religious path of life with faith in God. I accept that there is solace in the path of religious comfort. I hope there is appreciation that there is more than one way to face this issue.

I am not a philosopher by training, nor have the vast experience of dealing with dying people like some of my colleagues working in intensive care. My views are based on my interaction with people struggling to let go when appropriate. If there is a technical error in facts and figures, feel free to let me know.

I was surprised by the amount of literature, on line, in news magazines and many publications, when I started looking at various views before I wrote this book. It has not been possible to reference every resource, and authors. I thank everyone who have made contribution in this field, sociologists, psychologists, enthusiastic atheists, medical and care professionals. If have failed to refer you by name, accept my apologies.

Acknowledgements

I am grateful for many authors who have written fantastic chapters and quotes on this same subject. I do not intend to provide a list of bibliography, but a small list of inspirational books is attached at the end. I wish to express my thanks for all those authors. Many are great philosophers, leaders of the medical profession and gurus who have tried to solve the final mystery, the death. There are some questions still unanswered, and every step we take towards the truth will slowly one day lead us to acknowledgement and acceptance of reality.

I got many gifts from my late father; love of books and reading is one of them. His memories are guiding light in our life, his life is an inspiration to my writing career, and his end of life was a lesson and a motivation for this book.

My thanks and love to my little family, my wife Kanchan and my daughter Tejal, with whose support, this book has become a reality. I would like to express my profound sense of gratitude to my first teacher and my mother Sumitra.

I wish to thank Kindle Direct Publishing platform for providing me the opportunity to make a success of this book. I hope you enjoy the read.

- **Kishore Shanbhag.**

I BOW THEE,

Omnipresent, omnipotent, time immemorial and bright,

One who has no shape, size, smell, sound or in sight,

Both God and Death have much in common,

One is surety, other ambiguity and vain.

I bow thee, release me from this world's lust,

Grief, greed, anger, jealousy, mind filled with doubt,

O powerful, natural and magnificent end,

Let me finish this journey, with peace I blend.

Drive the ignorance away from the minds,

remove the concept of annihilation, hell and suffering,

let there be peace prevailing on this planet,

Om shanti hi, shanti hi, Shanti hi.

Pinnacle of Life

1 THE GREAT CERTAINTY

INTRODUCTION

"HUMAN history is marred with events of uncertain deaths. Conflicts, famine, floods, earthquake and even manmade weapons cause havoc in human life expectancy. However, in the post war era, public health interventions and medical advances, technology and better governance, and restrain in world order resulted in limiting the damages caused by conflict and disasters. Estimation of life expectancy is getting more accurate and figures are improving. Yes, there are increasing accidental deaths and suicides, but overall, there is more certainty to life than ever before in our history."

I wrote the lines above some time ago as an introduction to this book. I wanted to emphasize the fact that human life has become more predictable and there is some degree of certainty in most aspects of life. As I finally had the courage to start writing this book, everything changed. Today United Kingdom went into lockdown. Covid-19 is changing everything. The materialism, individualism, capitalism and even liberalism has to stand aside and make way. Life has been pushed back to the bottom layers of hierarchal needs. Almost inanimate, invisible virus changed the way of life so powerfully. Working in health service, I am well aware of shortcomings of human abilities. But nothing of this scale. Helplessness of individual and organisational strength is well exposed. But the human spirit, desire to help the fellow beings, the instinct to survive is powerful. I dedicate my writing to those who showed that consideration and compassion and to those sadly did not come through it.

Every crisis and struggle, open up new ideas. First, for me, it was a lesson. Change is possible, on a large scale. Human beings are capable of high degree of physical and mental adaptation. Nothing, no system, no belief is powerful enough to be permanent. We are all capable of adopting new ways of life, embrace new concept of living, challenge our beliefs. This can happen quickly and decisively. Second, there is uncertainty in life. Life events are as uncertain as they were, at any period of our existence. There is only one certainty. Yes, we do not know when, where and how. But with great certainty we can say, we all are going to die. *Life is finite.*

It may sound very rational and simple. Many of us know that simple truth. We are all mortals. That is true for all living organism. Perhaps except for humans? Our well-developed brain with its enormous capability of imagination, has created some degree of doubt and confusion in the matter. Afterlife in heaven, reincarnation, immortality, eternity and even preservation of physical remains have been discussed, believed and practiced. It is time to add some clarity, some certainty. *No if, no but, end of life is just that, end.*

KNOWLEDGE ABOUT DEATH

Death is cessation of life and dying is process that ends in death.

Apart from this we know nothing about death. The concept of death is very empty. Even experts on death know very little about it. There are two main reasons for this. No one has the experience of death who could come back from it and tell us about the experience. There is no near death. Death has not occurred until you have died and once you have died, there is no return to share your experience. Second, the end of life is beginning of emptiness, there is nothing to conceptualize. Hence no experience can be returned. Death unites us all, in the sense that we all are equally ignorant about it.

This appears to have been the view of the ancient Greek philosopher Epicurus: *"Death, the most terrifying of ills, is nothing to us, since so long as we exist, death is not with us; but when death comes, then we do not exist. It does not then concern either the living or the dead, since for the former, it is not, and the latter are no more. Our own death does not affect us while we're alive. The expectation or fear of death can affect us, but not death itself. Nor does it affect us when we're dead: nothing can affect us then"*. So, death, Epicurus thought, is nothing to us. It can never be bad to die. Not because the benefits of death outweigh the harms, but because death is powerless to do us any harm at all.

Death at least on the physical plane is clearly the terminating point from life and no one knows where exactly it merges into. Death is not separate from life, it is extension of life, the last act results in termination of the life process. Death however is real, and affects us all. It is definitive and decisive. It is simple termination of life. In any case of death, there is no subject to suffer harm. Because when death happens, the person ceases to exist, and there is no harm death can do to that person. This might sound as not compassionate to the near and dear one of the dead. It is very rational. All the people mourning, are alive, and if they do not acknowledge the true meaning of death, they will suffer from grief.

JAATASYA HI DHRUVO MRUTYU.

If you look at the sky late at night and notice the position of the stars, you will see that after a few hours they make the same movement as the Sun. Some stars will set in the west, other new ones will rise in the east, and all the stars will move following this pattern. Not all of them. The North star, or Polaris remains constant in its position. The explanation for this constant position of the North Star lies in celestial mechanics. This star is nearly in a direct line with the Earth's rotation axis in the sky. If we locate this star and note its position, we can come back in a few hours, days, or years and we will always find it in the same place. The other stars vary their position and will most likely be in other parts of the sky, but Polaris will not have moved. This useful aspect was basis for our ancestors in recognising directions in the darkness.

DHRUVA is the name for pole star in many Indian languages including Sanskrit. The word also used to imply meaning of fixed, firm, immovable, stable, permanent and constant. In addition to its meaning of perpetual, everlasting and eternal, dhruvam also means apex of a structure, summit of a mountain or a peak.

In Bhagavadgita, the Indian holy epic, chapter II verse 27, the word dhruvam is used to describe end of life as inevitable, sure and certain (Jatasya hi dhruvo mratyur – for one who is born, death is certain). Inspiration to this book is from application of all meanings of "dhruvam" to this line. Death as a stable, certain, inevitable sequence for anyone who is born, but also is the peak and pinnacle of the life process itself. North star can help you find directions in the darkest nights. You need to know to locate the position and recognise the star. Recognition of end of life is the same. Once you recognise and acknowledge the finitude of life, it will help you find the direction in life, even in the darkest hours. Like Dhruvam, death is the constant and certainty. Death is what gives life that exciting finish, the edge, the finale.

WHAT DEATH HAS DONE FOR US

Finitude of life is a potential motivator. In the end we will all succumb to that finitude, but we will try to keep it off for as long as possible. Great collective and individual human effort has gone into activities primarily designed to prevent death. Very survival of ancestors depended on their ability to feed themselves and protect from wild beasts. Invention of fire and agriculture were basic tools which prevented untimely death of many. Clothes to ware, safe places to sleep, easy access to basic life needs were all invented to prolong life and to improve quality of it.

Man's desire to live longer, or perhaps live forever, has driven him to invent great things. The science of medicine as a whole is a tool devised primarily to keep him alive as long as possible. Prevention, cure, regeneration, and prosthetic techniques have developed into a large industry and thrives on one's desire to live longer, healthier, looking better and able to enjoy life. No criticism for that. However, the medicine now thinks it is a failure of science, every time a person dies. Doctor has a problem in letting go a patient, at the appropriate time. I stress appropriate. In the end person will go as nature decides. But before that medicine is capable of doing significant damage to dignity and wellbeing of the person, meaning well, to prevent death.

But there is another side to it. Humanity as a whole with rare exceptions definitely fears it. Talking about death often leads to gloom and despondency. So little is known about the process, soon after death, it leaves a large vacuum for speculative description. Much of the gap in knowledge is filled by religious scriptures, cultural notes passed from generations to the next, with blind faith in the almighty power. None of these religious tones have been impartially scrutinised. Therefore, there is a total unflinching trust in what has been the only thing people believed for several generations. Until there is no substitute for this dependence, this trend is bound to continue. Every unknow thing has potential to create fear in human mind. Facts of death are largely unknown. So are facts about god and religion. The combination, dependency of one unknow over the other, has created an ever more fearful ambience. Enigma of death in a way is the root cause for the strangle hold of religion over the society and source for the need for invention of god.

So, the food we eat, clothes we ware, the doctor I see, and the scripture I read about the divine power, all were primarily invented to either prevent death or address the fear of it.

"No one wants to die. Even people who want to go to heaven don't want to die to get there. And yet death is the destination we all share. No one has ever escaped it. And that is as it should be, because death is very likely the single best invention of life. It is life's change agent. It clears out the old to make way for the new." (Steve Jobs, in his 2005 Commencement address to the graduating class at Stanford University)

Death may be an end to an individual. But as a species for the survival of the species, it is an absolute essential. Without the death and clearing out of the old and birth of the new, the genetic selection and survival of the fittest would be possible, there won't be any evolution, we would remain the chimps or same apes would rule the planet, depending on how you look at history. So, for nature recycling of individuals creating newer breeds and recycling elements to make them is an essential activity. That theory can apply to human species at intellectual level as well. Without recycling of individuals, world will be full of same thought, same genetics and same personalities. Every new generation comes with new set of idea, creating new skills, new genetic makeup and the life keeps evolving. People living longer and having less progeny can't be advantageous to the progress of the species. The alternation of death and birth, is the pulse beat for the species.

In the face of death, individually and collectively, we can achieve amazing things. There was dark clouds of depression and anxiety related to corona virus disease in United Kingdom in early 2020. The gloom spread to the economy, daily life, jobs, basic supplies and every possible civilised way of life was affected. Yet, the fear of death and shear determination to overcome it, collectively as a nation, made some impossible things happen. First Nightingale hospital in London was built in nine days, to care for patients with intensive care needs. The capacity to treat thousands needing intensive care beds and complex ventilatory process. In normal times I have waited a month for the health system to decide if I could have a piece of equipment or not. The "sense of time" death injects in humans and the power of it, is enormous.

WHY UNSOLVED MYSTERY

Human history has evidenced great philosophers and thinkers who thought about the mystery of death. With its unknowns, enigma and profound emotional events associated, one would think, death and issue of end of life would have been a fertile ground for thinkers, philosophers and maharishis. But most philosophers only tinkered around the reality of life. Either they did not have enough science to back them to move the body away from the soul, or the religious beliefs were so profound, they found it impossible to establish a clean end of life and soul, that is what death really is. However, we have been here before, and established, against prevailing belief that earth rotated round the sun, and we need to do this yet again.

I acknowledge that everyone does not want to understand intricacies of philosophy of life at death and life after death. However, I feel it is appropriate to inform the reader why we are in the dire state of understanding about death, at the present time. The historical context why so many philosophers refrained from admitting, explaining the simple fact, end of life is simply end of life, nothing after, nothing different. I am not a trained in philosophy, I am a surgeon. Some time ago I started reading "The story of Philosophy" by Will Durant. This book became a bridge between my ignorance and philosophy. I have taken some references from the book in discussion to follow.

The conflict of everlasting soul and the body as mortal vehicle goes back to Socratic philosophy. Plato wrote, we fear death because we are regrettably embodied. Every human has a body, and that body ushers in a host of anxieties and attachments, great and small. The body is the soul's prison and there is no escape from the body's needs until death. Since death, by definition, the separation of the soul from the body, the body makes knowing of the truth impossible. It constantly deceives us about what is "true" and "real". It is even a nagging impediment to learning. At the most general level, Plato consistently argues that a virtuous person will not fear his own death and a virtuous person will not fear or grieve the death of her family and friends. He also argued that a virtuous political organization will train its citizens not to fear death and will prohibit public manifestations of grief.

Aristotle came close to describing complete demise of the soul at the end of life. He was perhaps too worried about consequences of arguing against theological belief (Aristotle's subtle way of saving himself from anti-Macedonian hemlock? As described by Will Durant). Aristotle described the soul as entire vital principle of any organism, the sum of its powers and processes. The soul, as the sum of the powers of the body, can't exist without it. Aristotle gave the "soul" immortality by aligning with theologians, by suggesting the immortal soul is "pure thought" so pure that it is just like god, undefiled with action.

Voltaire muses how it's not known whether or not the soul lives on, in his letter to Frederick William, Prince of Prussia in November 1770, "It is very true that we do not know too well what the soul is, no one has ever seen it. All that we do know is that the eternal Lord of nature has given us the power of thinking, and of distinguishing virtue. It is not proved that this faculty survives our death, but the contrary is not proved either." Even if we do not know whether the soul lives on, Voltaire pragmatically advises that it is the best course of action to always do right, *"In the midst of all the doubts which we have discussed for four thousand years in four thousand ways, the safest course is to do nothing against one's conscience. With this secret, we can enjoy life and have nothing to fear from death."*

Confucius was criticized for avoiding discussions of death. He did not encourage his followers to seek eternal life, nor did he discuss death, gods, ghosts, and the unknown future or afterlife in detail. Confucius concluded that these issues were complicated and abstract, and that it was better to spend time solving the problems of the present life than to look into the unknown world of death and afterlife. He wanted to convey the importance of valuing the existing life and of leading a morally correct life.

Santayana wrote "why has man's conscience in the end invariably rebelled against naturalism and reverted in some form or other to a power of unforeseen? Perhaps because the soul is akin to the eternal and ideal, it is not content with that which is, and yearns for a better life; it is saddened by the thought of death, clings to the hope of some power that may make it permanent amid the surrounding flux."

I am keen to keep the discussion brief on reasons why the problem of death as permanent cessation of life was not stressed by philosophers historically. I have listed some examples. I will come to various religions and more philosophy, later in the book. However, we should view the thoughts of these thinkers in context of when and where they lived. It was difficult for many to write against religious beliefs of the time. Many did not have the concrete scientific evidence or knowledge of evolution and biology to justify the argument. It is however unfortunate that the scientific analysis was not only overlooked but even unjustifiably and ruthlessly condemned. Religious scholars did not see any necessity to tell the truth about death. It was convenient for all religions, for humans to believe in some form of continuum of existence. *No one has exploited the human fear of death more than the religions.*

DEFINING DEATH

Death is the cessation of life as indicated by the absence of blood circulation, respiration, pulse, and other vital functions. The accepted legal definition of death appears simple and firm on the surface.

As a child growing in rural India, I remember playing the role of a doctor in a school play. I was expected to touch a body to check it was cold, then hold the hand to check there was no pulse and shake my head and declare the person dead. I think that child play was accurate depiction of real life in rural India at that time. There were no ECG monitors, no brain electrical activity scans, no syringe drivers. Death was truly cessation of bodily functions.

Cardiopulmonary resuscitation (CPR) had resuscitated some people whose condition temporarily seemed to meet the criteria for death. I would call that a reversal of death process. Furthermore, life support systems had been devised to prolong respiration and other vital functions in people whose bodies could no longer maintain themselves. Advances were being made in transplanting cadaver organs to restore health and preserve the life of other people. If the person who was being maintained in a persistent vegetative state could be regarded as dead, then there was a chance for an organ transplantation procedure that might save another person's life. Existing definitions and rules, however, are still based on the determination of death as the absence of vital functions, and these functions were still operational, even though mediated by life support systems.

The term clinical death had some value. Usually this term referred to the cessation of cardiac function, as might occur during a medical procedure or a heart attack. A physician could make this determination quickly and then try CPR or other techniques in an effort to restore cardiac function. "Clinical death" was therefore a useful term because it acknowledged that one of the basic criteria for determining death applied to the situation, yet it did not stand in the way of resuscitation efforts.

Technological advances in monitoring the electrical activity of the brain made it possible to propose brain death as a credible concept, and it quickly found employment in attempting to limit the number and duration of persistent vegetative states while improving the opportunities for organ transplantation. The electrical activity of the brain would quickly become a crucial element in the emerging redefinition of death.

Actually, the advances in biomedical knowledge and technology have contributed greatly to the complexity that surrounds the concept and therefore the definition of death in the twenty-first century. Furthermore, the definition of death has become a crucial element in family, ethical, religious, legal, economic, and policy-making decisions.

THE TERMINOLOGY

Dighe, (also spelled dye) was a word in common usage in the fourteenth century at the time when Europe was devastated by the Black Death, a plague that annihilated perhaps as much as a third of the population. The Icelandic deyja and the Danish doe are cognates. Die and dying became established words in the English language during the plague years. Because of the sensitive nomenclature fostered in the early twentieth century by funeral directors, the literal usage of the term "dying" gave way to euphemisms such as "expire," "pass away," or "go to one's reward."

The word death is used in many ways. The context indicates the intended meaning in some instances, but it is not unusual for ambiguity. The three main ways word death is used are to describe an event, a condition or state of nonexistence of life. Death as an event. In this usage, death is something that happens. As an event, death occurs at a particular time and place and in a particular way. Death is an event that cuts off a life. Death as a condition is the crucial area in biomedical and bioethical controversy. Death is the irreversible condition in which an organism is incapable of carrying out the vital functions of life. It is not identical with death as an event because the focus here is on the specific signs that establish the cessation of life. Death as a state of nonexistence. In this sense, it can almost be said that death is what becomes of a person after death. Word dead, is used as a substitute.

End-of-life (EOL) has become another key term. Hospital protocols refer to treatment algorithm as end of life pathways. Unlike terminal illness, EOL calls attention to the many sources of potential concern and support. End of life, term is used in care profession as well as legal and financial sector. Other commonly used term at end of life is terminally ill or end phase of life. Some terminally ill people can continue with their family activities and careers, and look after much of their own care. People in the end-phase have lost much of their functional capacity and are likely to be receiving specialized care in the hospital or at home.

HOW DEATH AFFECTS OUR THINKING

Humans have ongoing conflict about believing and denial of death at the same time. We are able to imagine future and have knowledge that death is certain. But, deep in our mind, we have a strong desire not to believe this truth. This paradox ultimately drives everything we do, from choosing to attend temple, eat nutritious diet and go to the gym to motivating us to have homes, do research and write books. What we know about how death shapes behaviour in the real world? In the 1980s, psychologists became interested in how we deal with the potentially overwhelming anxiety and dread.

Ernest Becker asserted in his 1973 book "The denial of death", that humans, as intelligent animals, are able to grasp the inevitability of death. Becker criticised the previous writings of Sigmund Freud and Otto Rank. Becker replaces the Freudian preoccupation with sexuality with the fear of death as the primary motivation in human behaviour. Terror management theory, claims that humans embrace culturally constructed beliefs. We think that the world has meaning, and that our lives have value, in order to fend off what would otherwise be paralysing existential terror.

Researchers have found that, when reminded that we are going to die, we cling harder to foundational cultural beliefs and strive to boost our sense of self-worth. We also become more defensive of our beliefs and react with hostility to anything that threatens them. When reminded of death, we treat those who are similar to us in looks, political thinking, and religious beliefs more favourably. We become more intolerant towards people who do not share those similarities. We also become more nihilistic, drinking, smoking, shopping and eating in excess and we are less concerned about caring for the environment. Should everyone suddenly learn the date and means of their demise, society could become more racist, xenophobic, violent, warmongering, self-harming and environmentally destructive than it already is.

Researchers looking into a style of thinking called "death reflection" also have found that asking people to think not just about death in a general, abstract way, but to think about exactly how they will die and what impact their death will have on their families, elicits very different reactions. In that case, people become more altruistic. They are also more open to reflecting on the roles of both positive and negative events in shaping their lives.

Given these findings, learning about our death may lead us to focus more on life goals and social bonds rather than responding with knee-jerk insularity. This would especially be true "if we promote strategies that help us to accept death as part of life and integrate this knowledge into our daily choices and behaviour," says Eva Jonas, a psychology professor at the University of Salzburg. Knowing about the scarcity of life may increase the perception of life's value and promote tolerance and compassion and minimise defensive responses.

Palliative care patients, often experience two phases of thinking. First, they question the very premise of their diagnosis, asking if death is definitely imminently inescapable or whether it is something they can fight. After that, they contemplate how to make the most of the time they have left. Most fall into one of two categories. They either decide to put their whole energy and focus into doing everything they can to beat the illness, or they opt to reflect on their lives and spend as much time as possible with loved ones doing things that bring them happiness. Some people would probably decide not to fight their death, but spend time doing things that bring them joy.

SUMMARY

We have very little understanding of death. It is not opposite of life, but the integral part of it. There is nothing bad about death. Only thing death can do bad is, it will make you to miss rest of your life. You don't know what that missing bit is. So, mitigate that risk, don't miss the party, join it today when you are still here. In the world of humour, "If life is a joke, then death is a punchline!".

As a young parent, I used to tell my daughter, to motivate a sense of urgency in her, "time is money and money is everything". How wrong I was. Death awareness has great quality to bring perspective to life. I still retain my sense of urgency to do things. But my mantra has changed to "Time is everything and money is nothing".

LOOKING AT DEATH

Looking at life is like vision in the light,

you see the image on retina clear and bright.

Only if you think, the width of your spectrum is low,

One realises the sensory input is very slow.

Out there, vast space, in thoughts and in cosmos,

In beliefs, sensations and emotional feelings,

There is no particle, gravity or reflecting light.

Your limited sensory organ gives you no delight.

You need knowledge, thoughts, and imagination,

to enjoy the vast world of darkness and sublimation.

The pleasure is unlimited and contrast stark,

Looking at death is like looking in the dark.

2 A BUCKET LIST

WHY we struggle so badly facing with any issue related to death? Why a simple task of telling a patient about a condition with high or definitive risk of mortality is so difficult? Why as an individual, it is so upsetting for us to hear about a diagnosis of cancer? We all know that we are going to die, but when confronted with our own death, why it feels as if we never heard about it before?

The answer to all the question is same. We are unprepared. We are unprepared for the most certain thing in life. We do not think, talk, or reflect on our own death. It is almost masochistic, to not to know anything about it, not to do anything about it, then be stung by the arrival of it. Thinking about one's own mortality allows you to reflect on the process, prepare and deal with it. I am not asking you to welcome death, not even want it. Just be prepared. This is not a deal for the elderly or high risk. We are all mortals and we all need to prepare.

HOW do we prepare? Think death is a risk. We all, as individuals, institutions, business or a country know how to analyse and prepare for risks. Some better and some not so well. Better you are prepared, easier it is to deal with. Businesses spend lot of resources in dealing with risk management and probably have strategies we can adapt. So, may I say, a "business like" approach is needed to sole the risks posed by death.

Hence the bucket list. It is not list of the places you wish to see and things you want to experience before your death. Yes, that is an integral part of the list. But most important, a gradual process of changes in life activities, expectations, and transfer of power and responsibilities, enabling you that detachment in the end without struggle. There is no generalist approach, every individual has to work up a life path way suitable for their situation. I thought an outline of concepts would inspire.

MORTALITY RISK

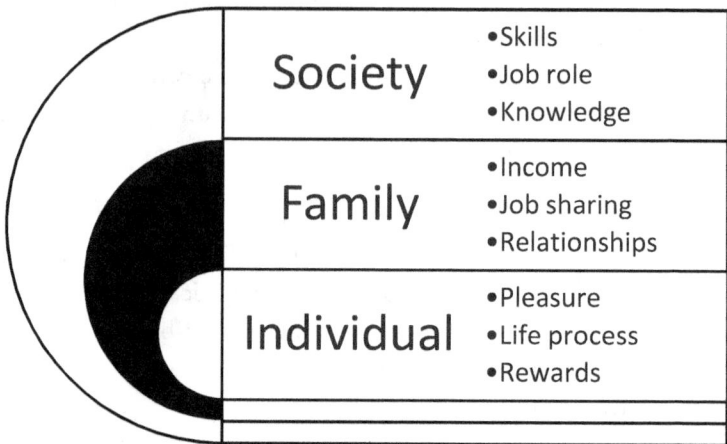

Illustration 1. Death of an individual can cause loss at various levels.

Any good risk management program will involve detailed analysis of identification of the risk and its causes, evaluation of the risk and defensive management or subjugation. Our lives involve uncertainties and risks. Sometimes, the uncertainty relates to the question of whether an event will occur. In case death, the event will definitely occur. The risk relates to the timing of the event. The risk management of individuals is strongly related to mortality because it determines the probabilities of dying and surviving. It is also related to words and concepts like life expectancy and to the measurement of the financial threats created by the life cycle risks.

The financial stages of life for adults can be categorized in the following seven periods: education phase, early career, career development, peak accumulation, pre-retirement, early retirement, and late retirement. A key element of risk management for individuals is life-cycle finance, which recognizes that as investors age, the fundamental nature of their total wealth, as do the risks that they face, vary. Individuals tend to follow a predictable pattern during their lifetimes: They invest in education early in life, embark on a career, start families, accumulate assets, fund growing household expenses, transition into retirement, and ultimately pass on wealth through bequests. In each of these life-cycle stages, the household faces unique goals and risks that require appropriate investment and risk management strategies.

A very individualised risk assessment therefore is needed to manage the risks associated with death. This planning also needs to be dynamic and should change with each significant life event and with progression of age to adapt the needs of the individual. There is a unit to measure risk of death! the MicroMort. The micromort was the brainchild of engineer Ronald A. Howard from Stanford University, who wanted an accurate unit to gauge the 'risk of death' we experience on a regular basis. Basically, a micromort stands for a one-in-a-million chance of death. So, if you have 2 micromorts, you have a two-in-a-million chance of dying.

UNEXPECTED DEATH

Premature or untimely death can be caused by trauma, homicide, suicide, infectious disease and many other conditions. Early onset heart conditions, cancers, and diabetes are increasingly cause of premature loss of death. War, famine, catastrophic natural events and epidemics can cause mass casualties. Infant death related to disease is another cause of premature death. I can't miss out a mention about the damage caused by a single epidemic of COVID-19, to every level of the social structure.

Every person should evaluate the risks associated with their own death on regular basis. Loss of life is a huge loss for the person dying, it brings to an end, all the joy of life, the passion, surprises, contacts and communication the person enjoyed all their life. But there will also be huge impact on other people due to your demise. Every individual has a human capital value, in addition to the earning potential, and social role. Sudden demise of a person creates a hole and vacuum in day to day life of people around, at family and friend group level as well as work place or organisational level. This vacuum needs to be filled. There will be significant amount of financial and social risks involved.

Obviously, the best strategy for managing the risk of premature death is the avoidance. Most premature deaths are avoidable. Last century has seen dramatic change in life expectancy due to implementation of death avoidance tools both medically and socially. Not speeding, wearing a helmet and not driving after drinking are avoidance tools related to vehicle accident related deaths. Life style changes, reduction in obesity, moderation in consumption of alcohol, cessation of smoking are all such social behaviours. Following health and safety guidance at work place, having preventive vaccination for hepatitis and flu help avoiding risk. Some risks can't be avoided and some people may choose to retain the risk of some activities. In case of death, by definition, the risk is not avoidable, but risk of premature death can be deferred. Every life activity has certain risk exposure and realisation that all risks can't be avoided, results in some risk retention. Such resulting risks, recognised early, can be shared, transferred or the loss from the risk can be reduced. This largely applies to the financial risk.

Financial risk of a premature death is mainly borne by the dependents of the deceased person because they relied on the income stream generated by the deceased. A premature death will be defined as dying prior to a certain age, commonly the expected retirement age. The death of a person typically results in a variety of losses: the direct loss is to the dying person because the person is unable to continue enjoying what he or she was doing and still wished to do. Family members and friends suffer a psychological and emotional loss from the disappearance of their loved one. However, the economic loss is mainly felt by people who depended financially on the deceased person (e.g., spouse, children, parents) and who lost the future income that would have been earned if the person had not died. Of course, there are also business interests that could be damaged; for example, the employing firm that lost a key person who held particularly important know-how or who had exceptionally important and strong ties with suppliers, customers, or regulators. Another common type of loss is that of a partnership that lost a key partner, a situation that may endanger the continuation of the business.

The term premature death, which is sometimes referred to as mortality risk, relates to the death of an individual earlier than anticipated whose future earnings, or human capital, were expected to help pay for financial needs and aspirations of the individual's family. These needs include funding day-to-day living expenses, such as food, housing, and transportation, as well as paying off debts, saving for a child's education, and providing for a comfortable retirement for the surviving spouse. An individual's death may also lead to a reduction in the income of the surviving spouse because some family responsibilities of the deceased individual must now be performed by the surviving spouse. For a young family, the effect can be especially tragic because the increase in household lifestyle that might have accompanied the career of the deceased may never occur.

A risk to consumption needs also occurs if a non-earning member of the family dies. The loss can be estimated as the discounted value of the services provided by the deceased family member plus any out-of-pocket death expenses. If a household's primary caregiver dies, the rest of the family can help with that member's responsibilities, but often additional, paid help is required to replace the primary caregiver's duties. This scenario will mean a dramatic change in lifestyle, compounding the incalculable emotional effect of the death. It could even have a negative impact on the career of the surviving spouse, who may feel drained by the added responsibilities.

Besides the obvious reduction in human capital that the death of an income earner represents, there are also effects on financial capital. Death expenses including funeral and burial, transition expenses, estate settlement expenses, and the possible need for training or education for the surviving spouse are among the financial costs that may be incurred.

Life insurance provides a hedge against the risk of the premature death of an earner. A family's need for life insurance is related to the risk of the loss of the future earning power of an individual less the expected future spending of that individual. In each case, the risk associated with premature death can be mitigated by transferring the risk to a third party by purchasing life insurance. The optimal amount of insurance to purchase is a function of both the expenses of the insurance hedge and the magnitude of the difference in expected lifetime utility with and without that family member. The optimal amount of life insurance for an individual will vary based on a number of factors. Some individuals with no dependents or bequest goals may not need any insurance, whereas an individual with young children and a non-working spouse may need a significant amount of life insurance. In this section, we outline some of the key considerations to use when determining how much life insurance to purchase.

FACILITATING GOOD DEATH

The risk of dying in old age is mainly borne by the person who is dying. The needs of finance, care and dependency and cost of medical management are major considerations. Individuals have a finite but unknown lifespan. The efficient allocation of financial resources across an unknown lifespan is a planning challenge because consumption smoothing requires the allocation of available financial resources across an expected time frame. Humans may plan to spread their resources based on an average lifetime, but this strategy exposes them to the risk of outliving their assets in old age. One efficient strategy is to pool the risk of an unknown lifespan across individuals through the use of an annuity.

Annuities have existed in a variety of forms for thousands of years. The Romans sold a financial instrument called an "annua" that returned a fixed yearly payment, either for life or for a specified period, in return for a lump sum payment. Even today, annuities remain popular risk management tool, especially for older individuals and retirees who want to mitigate the risk associated with outliving their assets (i.e., longevity risk). Annuities are generally purchased from an insurance company; however, government pensions and pay out from employer pension plans are also technically annuities.

DYING TOO LATE – RISK MITIGATION

The late retirement phase is especially unpredictable because the exact length of retirement is unknown. This uncertainty about longevity for a specific individual is known as longevity risk, which is the risk that retirement could be very short or very long. Physical activity typically declines during this phase, as does mobility. Although many individuals live comfortably and are in good health until their final days, others experience a long series of physical problems that can deplete financial asset reserves. Cognitive decline can present a risk of financial mistakes, which may be hedged through the participation of a trusted financial adviser or through the use of annuities.

Two additional concerns may be appropriate to any financial stage. First, depending on the family situation, the need to provide for long-term health care may become apparent. Second, some people may need to devote resources to care for parents or a disabled child for an extended period of time. An extended retirement period may deplete the retiree's resources to the point at which income and financial assets are insufficient to meet post-retirement consumption needs. A common question posed to financial planners is, "How much money do I need to have when I retire?" The answer is dependent on the lifespan of the individual, and longevity is a key variable that can only, at best, be estimated. Other important variables include the nominal rate of return on the portfolio, the rate of inflation, additional sources of income (and whether those sources are adjusted for inflation), and the level of spending. Determining how large a fund an individual will actually have at retirement depends on the amount and timing of contributions, the nominal rate of return, and the amount of time until retirement.

Dying too late has more implications than just running out of finances. Ageing is a cumulative process and some degree of incapacity lack of cognitive ability and dependency will develop in the process. This can lead to personality changes, behavioural changes in the person in addition to demanding medical and social care needs.

ARS MORIENDI

In the wake of the Black Death, priests, the cultural guarantors of salvation through the administration of last rites became a scarce commodity. Without enough priests to attend to the dying, the newly minted printing press offered a contemporary solution for salvation, allowing pamphlets containing prayers and penances to be easily producible and distributable. It was during this time of 15th century innovation and scarcity that the Latin texts known as Ars Moriendi began circulating European households. Ars Moriendi, literally "The Art of Dying," offered advice on how to die well according to the Christian ideals of the time.

The science of dying is being redefined. The art of dying may also be changing in our culture, where we can learn to live well not in spite of death but because of it. With a new narrative that demystifies death, we see that the end of life dignity sought out in hospices and hospitals may in fact lie in a life well lived. As Sherwin Nuland expertly wrote, *"Ars moriendi as ars vivendi: The art of dying is the art of living. The honesty and grace of the years of life that are ending is the real measure of how we die. It is not in the last weeks or days that we compose the message that will be remembered, but in all the decades that preceded them."* In the fifteenth and sixteenth centuries the Ars moriendi, that is, art offering aid to the dying and instruction to the living, represented an additional theme used by artists. Ars moriendi focused on the moment of death and functioned as a kind of handbook. Typically, they included ten images with text portraying the five temptations confronting the dying person, and five corresponding inspirations that enabled repentance and final reconciliation. Ars Moriendi in the new technological medicalised death is about choosing, and making options clear.

One example of choosing well is the decision regarding medical intervention. Hospital doctors are trained to save life and treat any death as failure, so everything is done to prolong life. Many people use up their life savings in the last six months of their lives on ultimately futile medical interventions. Some interventions are done simply to ensure there is no change in the health condition, like daily blood tests on the hospital wards. It is time for person to ask questions, even a small intervention like blood test, if it really going to change that management of the situation person is in. Then it applies to bigger decisions, whether to have a surgery or not, to have chemotherapy to prolong life at reduced quality of life or to have better quality of life for shorter period.

As quality of life is a fundamental decisive factor, so is quality of death anticipated. Would the proposed treatment reduce the discomfort when I eventually die? Will the course of treatment change the mode of death?

Example : an untreated cancer may grow to cause internal bleeding and cause sudden death, harsh it may sound, some patients, when explained carefully, may choose to have that death. Patient will be in a prearranged care package, when the bleed occurs, there will be ready prescription to administer a sedative to keep patient calm and pass away. No attempt will be made to stop bleeding or enhance other functions like oxygen saturation etc. As opposed to this patient may choose to have chemo radio therapy on the same tumour mass, which will reduce its size and reduce risk of bleeding. However, it is not curable and tumour cells may spread through the body, eventually use up patient's nutrition, muscle mass and death may result from cachexia and malnutrition. It may appear that the later case, death is more planned, delayed and slow, many patients prefer the death without going through the palliative chemo radio therapy. It is the personal preference.

Codes and medical ethics explicitly indicate the importance of respecting patients' rights, goals and values, as well as good communication, advance care planning, and recognising when continuing treatment is more harmful than beneficial.

HANGING UP YOUR BOOTS – ASHRAM OF VANAPRASTHA

According to ancient Hindu philosophy a person's life was broadly categorised into four stages called ashrams. The first stage was the Brahmacharya, followed by Grihastha, Vanaprastha and Sannyasa. These ashrama dharmas regulated the life of the people living in the ancient societies and guided them with certain standards of behaviour to be observed during each stage of life. Those were the rules of living of those times which people observed.

The Brahmacharya Ashrama provided the guidelines for childhood and adolescent stage and certain basic values were to be adhered to. These values had some basic objectives — to train the children, to exercise control over the sense organs, that were the root cause of all undesirable behaviour. Thus, it offered a prescription for a healthy mind-body coordination and disciplined development to prepare for an ideal citizen.

The Grihastha Ashrama offered the prescription for a healthy family life. It provided for the pleasures of worldly life in a righteous manner. From marriage to procreation, from industry and entrepreneurship to wealth and prosperity, that was necessary to ensure the progress of society and the world. The third ashrama that was the Vanaprastha, which people entered after fulfilling all duties of the family life —that is from bringing up a family to rearing children and then preparing them for facing the world and shoulder the responsibilities of a family life.

Thus, it was like passing the mantle in a relay providing both continuity and change. This was the gateway to the final stage, the Sannyasa, which could lead to moksha or liberation after living a full life. It was the ashrama dharma that gave a systematic prescription to ideal living and had a very rational basis for ensuring order in society. Though for many today, this would appear to be a puritan and traditional approach for displaced from the norms of modern living, it did have the ingredients of the idealistic modern approach. The purpose of describing the life into four stages was to ensure that people played their part in this world and made way for the future generation.

It is against this backdrop that the significance of the Vanaprastha stage has to be understood. It was something like succession planning, a popular management jargon of the corporate world.

Passing the mantle to somebody after preparing him or her to shoulder those responsibilities was the right approach for a healthy society where opportunities were not denied. The biggest problem of the modern living is that people never realise the importance of Vanaprastha. Hanging the boots is a popular phrase that explains the significance of Vanaprastha. It is difficult to time the stage of hanging the boots. When to pave way for next generation is a difficult question to answer in the modern times when people just don't want to give up their power and self.

YOUNG people live in future and as you get older, you start living in the past. When those who have striven for wealth, name, and fame, retire from active life, they feel emptiness. Their worldly achievements no longer seem attractive. They feel a strong craving for peace and true joy. Most of these people have enjoyed enough worldly life and public life; they have fulfilled their duties towards family and society. However, they feel emptiness within. How do they address this emptiness? Those having spiritual aspiration from their youth may try to get involved in activities with their chosen organization, where their spiritual quest can flourish. When such activities are performed without attachment the aspirant will gain true joy and fulfilment. Some try to use their knowledge and experience in activities benefiting society at large, without seeking personal gain. Such selfless work will give them inner joy and fulfilment. Those who are well-to do, having adequate finances and shelter and good health, have the freedom to live their life in their own way, and may try to find joy and peace by engaging themselves in activities of their choice, like traveling, socializing with their friends, or spending occasional quality time in solitude. Such people will also find inner joy and fulfilment. Yet others will choose to spend lots of time in reading, writing, researching, creating new things, painting, music, dancing, and other art-related activities and find joy and fulfilment in those things.

As a vanaprastha there will be little for others to identify with, so you will have to rely largely on yourself to explain your position and how you want people to interact with you. An intelligent person realizes that one day everything material will be lost. It is all taken away, or rather we are taken away from all of it. The more detachment, the less the pain. The more knowledge, the more detachment. Understanding that we are not controllers relieves us from the fear of failure. We have a right to perform our duty but we are not entitled to the results. This brings detachment.

DECLUTTERING – THE SWEDISH "DOSTADNING"

The word dostadning, is hybrid Swedish word meaning death and cleaning. Basically, it implies a form of decluttering, but with a view of death of the owner of the possessions in mind. The elderly and their families put their affairs in order. As we live longer, we tend to accumulate more stuff. And unlike Egyptians of the gone era, we no longer believe that we may need some of our possessions for our afterlife. Dostadning advocates the practice of proactive clearing out of possessions before death, or at least put them in order. A way of death planning.

The idea is to have less burden passed on to your family when you eventually die. It also allows you to spend some time with your possessions, think and decide the appropriate disposal of everything as you see fit. Perhaps, your family members may not value things as you would for a particular item. It will also allow you to decide what you would like to hang on to, until your death. The process saves your family lot of time and stress.

This is not a form of will making or distribution of your wealth. It is more of a tidy up. Exact practice or the wording is less important. But as an activity, I think it will be much appreciated by the society as a whole, and family in particular.

Some-one somewhere might need your stuff more than your family. Charitable donations are desperately needed to support good causes. This process need not just apply to your furniture, books and clothes. What about the collection of digital music? The albums, the art collection, gift from your near and dear ones you kept as memory but really never used. The process will also reduce the need for packing and storage and eventual disposal of items.

There are lot of other things, most of it involve serious decluttering and paperwork, to take care of matters before you go, and while it may seem scary, complicated or just plain depressing, planning for death is an essential part of life, whether you expect to pass soon or are simply taking care of things just in case. What better legacy to leave behind a clean cupboard, to ease the burden at the time of bereavement?

DEATH AWARENESS

Death awareness is simply that. The awareness of death. The awareness of the fact that someday, we will all die. And the awareness that death is not just something that takes place in the faraway future, but that it is happening always, everywhere, all around us, right now. One of the objectives of this book is to raise death awareness: to encourage people to have conversations about death and dying, and by doing so, hopefully making them less afraid of it. Death awareness increases your appreciation of life. The finite nature of life is due to unpredictability of death, and this makes existence of life precious. Constant threat of death, no matter what age, makes living more exciting. Contemplating death could be an uplifting experience.

No one wants to be reminded of own mortality. As a society, have learned to ignore death. Deep down inside, all of us know death is inevitable. But instead of exploring the reality, we turn try to look as far from it as possible. We keep ourselves busy to ignore death. What really scares us is the gap, between the unknow of death and the busy material world we cover ourselves in. We are uncomfortable in situations when we are faced with death. Like dealing with a terminally ill family member and figuring out what you can do for them. Arranging or even just attending a funeral. Comforting someone facing bereavement. These are the most important moments in life, and for the most part we do not deal with them well.

When you look at the history of how we cope with death, you will see that our death rituals have "evolved" a lot. Whether this is a good thing or not, they have certainly changed drastically. Where we used to tend to our deceased loved ones ourselves and for example wash and dress the body, we now distance ourselves from any physical contact through the medical customs that have been pre-arranged for us, to which we often simply give in because we don't know any better. Death has been removed away from the sight of the society, handled, sanitised and packaged in business of hospitals and care homes. This has further reduced exposure of death and awareness day to day life.

We can't normalize death but we can familiarize with it. The past few years a lot of new initiatives have been set up to improve death awareness. In America, The Order of the Good Death founded by Caitlin Doughty has kick-started the death-positive movement by spreading knowledge on how to make death an integrated part of life. The concept of Death Cafe's which are now taking place all over the world: real life meet-ups to discuss mortality and grief over tea and cake.

Contemporary medicine has enabled us make choices related to our death. Certainly, there is some assurance that most deaths are pain free and serene in historical comparison. Most times it is possible for person and family to make a choice where the death should occur and what interventions if any should be continued until time of death. People do not simply "die", death can be arranged to happen in a biologically and even perhaps socially acceptable way.

Death can strike without any notice. My heart goes to victims of COVID -19 whose demise came with a shock and circumstances of such short period of changes. Unprecedented it is, but I reiterate the feeing, there is no better time to start becoming death aware. Unanticipated death or death after a very short illness accounts for significant proportion of total morbidities.

DENUNCIATION – "SANYASA"

Death is about losing "I"and "Me". In very individualistic societies, the "I" centered personalities will have difficulty in accepting death.

A gradual detachment therefore necessary to facilitate death. More stronger the bondage to the "I", more difficult the demise. We use our body towards pleasure, emotions, libido and create sense of self identity. But these things are limited and undermined by material aspect of the body, which ultimately will decay. Denunciation is a way of gradual detachment of self from the material world.

In Hinduism sanyasa means giving up all desires, and thereby freeing the mind from all attachments and expectations. A Sanyasi becomes mentally free from everything that holds him in control, before becoming free from the mortal life itself. Physical and mental freedom precedes spiritual freedom through the act of renunciation. We may define a Sanyasi as the one who lives without intentions and expectations and who makes no deliberate effort to be or to have anything.

The Bhagavadgita goes a step further and declares that true denunciation (sanyasa) is giving up desires and desire for the fruit of actions rather than giving up actions themselves. In other words, a Sanyasa does not have to live in the forests or in a monastery to achieve liberation. He can live in the world and yet practice sanyasa by living selflessly. He can perform his duties without desires.

Sanyasa is effortless and aimless living, or living without purpose, with inner self as a guide. It is the negation of life to break the habits of the mind and body and set oneself free from the delusion and ignorance caused by the field of Maya.

A sanyasi has to remain unattached to himself and to everything here and hereafter, be it an idea, thought, opinion, belief, doctrine, religion, a god or a goddess. He cannot depend upon anyone or anything, has to give up all the urge to control or regulate his life or that of others, and live as if he does not exist and does not matter. In other words, he has to become empty like space and insignificant like a fallen, autumn leaf on the edge of life as if he is already dead and his presence or absence would not cause any observable or noticeable difference to the world.

True denunciation is therefore an attitude of indifference, equanimity or sameness. It is a way of life, in which the renunciant sets aside his desires and expectations to let go off all intentional effort and compulsive planning. He lets things happen, identifying himself with his essential nature and true Self.

Denunciation is one of the fundamental pillars of Gautama Buddha's teaching. Suffering arises from clinging to impermanent things. Life is filled with pain and misery because of fundamental ignorance of reality, humans constantly desire for death not to occur.

PLANNING AHEAD

Humans have an instinctive desire to go on living. We experience this as desires for food, activity, learning, etc. We feel attachments to loved ones, such as family members and friends, and even to pets, and we do not want to leave them. We do not so much decide to go on living, as find ourselves doing it automatically. Robert Frost said, "In three words I can sum up everything I have learned about life: It goes on." Even in difficult times, it is our nature to hold on for better times.

But nothing stops us from planning ahead. Planning ahead means thinking about what is important, and what is not. It also means talking about this with those close to us. Even though we think we know what someone else thinks and believes, we really do not know until we ask. You cannot read other people's minds.

What can you plan ahead? Everything. Things you can plan for yourself before you die, the holiday you always had in mind, that book you wanted to write and the money you wanted to donate. Get them out of the way. Things you can plan for the event of your death, where when and how you wish to die if the events permit this to happen, or perhaps most importantly how you don't want it to happen. Then perhaps you can have some say in what happens after your death. Legacy, a Will, estate planning, funeral and good bye, how you want to be remembered, list is long and variable for every individual.

When we think about the last part of our own or someone else's life, consider these questions, What makes life worth living? What would make life definitely not worth living? What might at first seem like too much to put up with, but then might seem manageable after getting used to the situation and learning how to deal with it? If I knew life was coming to an end, what would be comforting and make dying feel safe? What, in that situation, would I most want to avoid? Knowing what really matters to you is worth considering. How important is being able to talk with people, engaging in daily activities, physical comfort or general alertness to you? What comes to mind when you think about the burden of care on others, being at home, or not being there? How much distress is it worth in order to live another month? And what medical procedures are not worth enduring? From your perspective, what is the best way for a person to die, and how important is it to you to be in control of how you live and how you die? Whose opinion should be sought in making choices about the care received when an illness has progressed to an advanced stage?

SUMMARY

I have discussed risk management approach to loss occurring from dying using financial mitigation as an example. Practical measures are needed for subjugation of risk. Gradual changes in your life activities should be aimed at achieving detachment from earthly possessions and powers. This facilitates eventual good bye. You are in control of most eventualities and they can be accomplished if you plan ahead.

INTO EMPTINESS

Galloping round the world, picking up the speed

You have come close to the escape velocity.

Journey through the path, across the land scape,

You are nearing the summit of mountain of life.

Friction from roughness of life, absorbing enough heat

You are closing in on boiling point.

Climbing step after step, you have achieved enough height,

When you look back, you find only little dots.

Your eyes have been looking out at life, far and future,

Now see from your mind, inside the lobe below the suture,

It is time to release into space, sublimate, climb to the top,

Go where you came from, into emptiness, zero behind the one.

3 IT IS YOUR CHOICE

Religious belief provides solace to the dying person and his family. It is known that people with religious beliefs suffer less anxiety and fear about death. You have a choice, take solace in ignorance or explore the truth. Where your experience and religion contradict, then it is up to you to investigate the conflict. Of course, you can choose to ignore the conflict altogether. However, a well-informed choice is always preferable to the blind belief

SUCH THING AS GOOD DEATH

Is there such thing? Every society in history had their own version of good death. Contemporary representation of good death is often associated with terms like dignity, control, painless and peaceful. Largely it is the perspective of the family and the dying, what decides a death was good or not. The deciding factors include the timing of death, place of death, manner of death, degree of medicalisation and control of individual over the process. I have discussed various options under each category. Remember, the choice is yours and there is no right option!

We also turn to doctors and medical care in the hope that the right physician, medication, treatment, or surgical procedure will make death optional rather than inevitable. But death, of course can't be made optional, even with the finest medical care or the most resolute denial of its existence. And in the meantime, our discomfort with death causes us to spend little or no time getting ready – emotionally, spiritually, or practically – for that inevitable day when our life will end. As a result, death too often catches us unprepared emotionally, spiritually and practically. But it doesn't have to be that way. Rather than spending time and energy avoiding and denying death, it is prudent, practical, and, in my opinion, healthier to put time and energy into getting ready for death.

Briefly, try and enlist what it means by good death to you?

1. A good death should occur after a long but healthy life. Of course, in death can happen in the middle of a long life! The question however is how long is long. What is the age we call a ripe age? And you might want to live few more years after the ripe age. Some of you really feel Pro-Life and want to get very best of the life till the last possible, even if it is a bit uncomfortable.
2. Some of us might want a few weeks or months Good death should give you some notice? Or really? to tidy up matters after a terminal illness diagnosis. Others might want a quick surprise demise. A cancer death gives you some notice, but a surprise cardiac arrest, you may not have that choice.
3. A good death should be entirely painless and comfortable. But what should make it comfortable and how slowly you want to fade away? Absence of pain and discomfort can be induced by appropriate use of medication the term used is "syringe driver induced oblivion". Some chronic debilitation like liver cirrhosis can cause gradual incapacitation leading to death.
4. Some may prefer death to occur away from sight of family and others wish to die surrounded by the friend and family, perhaps in familiar environment like own home.
5. Some may want to die of old age and others may wish to die for a cause like on a battlefield, fighting Corona Virus, on a crusade or for a religion manipulated

martyrdom. Some might want to mitigate all the losses of their death, with the potential spiritual gains.
6. No death is a good death, if you don't accept it. You can't accept death if you are not aware and prepared. And you can't be prepared, unless you had good life. So, a good life is a precursor to a good death.
7. God death causes least discomfort for those you have left behind. Again, there are strategies to achieve this you can develop.
8. Last, a person may qualify a good death according to personal religious or cultural belief or wishes. This may include last rites likes the holy water from Ganges, presence of a priest or chanting or verses from Quran. It could be physicality of death like dying on the floor or dying in your home country.

THERE IS ALWAYS HOPE

Hope is the only thing what keeps us going. There should always be hope. Without hope there is hopelessness, despair. Suffering and loss are exaggerated in absence of hope. In time of greatest personal loss, what kind of hope should we cling to? Hope based on incorrect facts lead to wrong expectations and often leads to disappointment and distress. Out of kindness or cowardness, many occasions we give dying person and their families false sense of hope. It may be from an article in leading newspaper talking about new gene therapy promising cure to a person with neurological disease. It may be from a medical professional, going bit soft on the significance of the findings of a new scan to a cancer patient. Without acknowledgement of true facts, we live in hope of that slightest chance, that one day science or medical advancement will bail us out.

False hope can lead to intemperate choices and flawed decision making. True hope takes into account the real threats that exist and seeks to navigate the best path around them. (Anatomy of hope – Jerome Groopman). At least in part, I feel the false hope created by the religion about afterlife allows the young and vulnerable to be exploited by the religious extremists. The lure of afterlife rewards is used to brainwash young people to agree to sacrifice their own life. Like fear, hope is a powerful emotion, in times of dire need, it is human tendency to clutch any straw. It should be the mission of the modern religion to eradicate false sense of hope.

There can be hope, and there should always be hope. Hope may not change the outcome, but it can help us to cope with the journey or even enjoy it. The road built on hope is always more pleasant to the traveler. So, what kind of hope should we give to the dying person or their loved one? The assurance of peace and painless passing as a start. To attend to their anxiety, fear, the fact that we will support their wishes. This is the true kindness, to facilitate the end of the journey in exactly the way the person wanted it to be. Reassurance that we will be there to support the family. The hope that tomorrow will be as beautiful as today and we will always cherish the memories. There is no worm in the core, only seeds of hope. Hopes of a new dawn or a spring. Replenishing lost lives with new life is nature's way of reincarnation.

TIMING OF DEATH

We control most things in our life, obviously no one can control events of nature, but surely, we can influence it. We have birth control, which is advertised everywhere but discussion of controlled end of life upsets people. Everyone should have the right to choose when, where and how they wish to die. They may not to wish to act on it or may not have the opportunity to facilitate it, but at least you can think about it. Across the whole Western world, there is increasing public debate about the exercise of individual control over the timing and manner of death. More and more people, especially in old age, seem to be trying to take control over the way in which they die, as we see in practices such as advance directives, living wills, requests for assisted dying. Despite the absence of a serious medical disease, people want to have the option to choose death in anticipation of age-related deterioration and expected suffering.

Before we plan to respond to this demand in an ethical way, we need to understand why there is such demand, can we address the issue why people feel that way. I feel death anxiety and social attitude towards old age and dying is contributing to this problem. Many elderly people have lost their traditional place in the society, where they were valued as law makers, educators, intermediaries in disputes, etc. A general respectful term collectively we refer as the "tribal elderly" as we live all our life in self-centered, individualistic, egocentric life style, when old age approaches us, we struggle to make necessary adaptations to our life style. In the final chapter I will refer this to as "deciding your own life pathway". When people fail to recognise their own value in the society, they might incline to reach the conclusion that their life is no longer worth living. They also increasingly wish to avoid demeaning decline and suffering by a pre-emptive death.

No one wants to think about death due to sense of loss attached to it. Also, people are worried about the manner of actual death, worries about what comes after death, and significantly the effect it may have on near and dear ones. Fear of the unknown is a factor. Living, some time, may not make sense, but dying without reason makes no sense at all. Dignity, control and independence, at least a degree of it, is needed to keep living. I have discussed issues of assisted dying, suicide and euthanasia later in the chapter.

There is some research to suggest people can, some degree control time of their death. Researchers found that, on average, people were 14 per cent more likely to die on their birthday than any other day. The study only looked at natural causes of death, so the statistical anomaly couldn't be confounded by other things that might be brought on by people celebrating excessively, for example. Still, heart attacks rose 18.6 per cent on birthdays, strokes by 21.5 per cent. Several studies since the 1980s have found strange patterns in mortality statistics. One found that death rates among Jewish men dropped by 25 per cent before Passover, an event in which they take a lead role. Similarly, researchers looking at death rates in Chinese women found a 35 per cent decrease in the days leading up to the Harvest Moon festival. In both cases, there was a corresponding peak in death rates in the days after the holidays.

The decision to voluntarily stop eating and drinking at the end of life is a choice a person may make for more than one reason. Certainly, the decision may be made with the intent to hasten the dying process. But the underlying reasons may go deeper than this. Most people are not hungry at the end of their lives. In this setting, eating may be seen as an unnecessary discomfort while prolonging the discomfort of the underlying disease. The end result of not eating is that people can feel as though they are taking control at the end of their lives. What this means is that there might be a coherent desire for immortality after all. This is because desiring immortality might not simply be about having a desire to live forever. It might instead be a desire to control when we ourselves will die, choosing to end it all only when, and not before, we ourselves are ready.

Indeed, such a possibility is depicted in the ancient Sanskrit epic *Mahabharata*, where the great warrior Bhishma is granted the boon of 'death upon desire'. Bhishma cannot die until he wishes to die. He falls in the battle incapacitated on a bed of arrows. When so incapacitated, Bhishma is not yet ready to die. He elects first to lie on the field of battle and pass on his wisdom, until he has decided that the time has come for him to depart. Bhishma prepares himself for death, and when he is ready, draws his life to a close. This capacity for 'death upon desire' is presented in the *Mahabharata* explicitly as a boon. And the contrast with immortality as being somehow unable to die is clear. Had Bhishma been incapacitated and unable to die on the bed of arrows due to immortality, we could interpret immortality as a curse. Bhishma' s boon seems coherent as something we might want for ourselves. It would eradicate fears of dying before we are ready, at the same time as preserving a capacity to call it quits when we've had enough.

In the Greek legend, handsome young Tithonus was kidnapped by Eos, goddess of dawn. Eos fell in love with Tithonus and makes him immortal like her, but forgot to get him eternal youth. As he aged, Tithonus become demented, and weak. Eos turned him into a Cicada, alive forever but calling for death. By postponing death, we develop risk of debilitating illness and dementia. By using technology, by keeping people alive for longer, we are only increasing risk of chronic sickness. The result of preventive medicine and lifestyle paradoxically resulting in elderly care homes filled with anxiety and depression. More people suffer from cancer and Alzheimer's than any other generations before.

Of course, the harsh reality is that most of us will find that death comes either 'too early or too late'. Too early, if we are not yet ready to go. Too late, if we've gotten to the point where life is already not worth living anymore. Indeed, we hardly need philosophers to convince us that, for many people, there are fates worse than death: assisted dying clinics in countries such as Switzerland demonstrate that many people will choose to die rather than carry on in gross physical pain or continued indignity, especially when there is no prospect of recovery. It is a striking feature, however, of most societies that they deny people the choice to die at the very point when they most rationally desire it.

Immortality is, an impossible fantasy hence it cannot be a genuine solution. Nonetheless, the reason immortality endures in popular imagination is that it addresses something about our attitudes towards death. We are not simply afraid of death, we also resent it. Death is more complicated than it appears. Most of us think it's a bad thing to die. There are, of course, exceptions. Some people actively want to die. They might be unbearably lonely, or in chronic pain, or gradually sliding into senile dementia that will destroy their intellect without remainder. And there might be no prospect of improvement. They wake up every morning disappointed to find that they haven't died in their sleep. In these cases, it might be better to die than to continue a life not worth living. But most of the time death is unwelcome, and we do all we can to avoid it.

MEDICALISATION OF DEATH

Medicine is all about curing disease, and saving and preserving life. Medicine's traditional ethic has been to benefit patients by treating them and not giving up. Doctors are trained to make people better, or else keep them alive and have difficulty some times to let go. Life is sacred and medicine views every death as a failure of the science of medicine. The potential harms in this singular pursuit have been difficult for the profession to acknowledge, in part because being responsible for death has been regarded as a far greater harm.

Intense care units have become specialised mass units of keeping people alive. I will not go into medical details of the practices, but it is sufficient to say that unless actively indicated by the patient, the medical profession has habit of going heroically too far to keep patient somehow alive. In many circumstances it is rewarding and greatly appreciated by the patients and family, but there should be a recognition that it may not be appropriate to every patient and there should be a choice. The choice for the patient. During the COVID-19 pandemic, over stretched intensive care units had to develop an algorithm, a triage system to decide which patient will receive critical care. Metrics used were based on likely prognostic factors, age, frailty and underlying conditions. Can such system including patient choice be used in normal working practice to avoid unnecessary medicalisation of the end of life? The great difficulty in talking about death, is in recognising the point at which treatment harms begin, to outweigh benefits. Because this has been a matter of professional conundrum for a significant time, the calls for change have not produced immediate results. Some super-specialists, are focused on the organ of their specialty, the heart, the kidney, the brain and so forth, and don't see the bigger picture.

These super specialists (Organologists) know they can bring about improvements in organ function, and so doing they feel there is no need to talk about death. Indeed, to do so would imply to the patient that you have lost hope, and medicine traditionally is the bringer of hope. Cancer specialist focus on the bit of tissue which has cancer, how to remove it, and what to put in its place. The liver specialist tries and see if they can decompensate the effects of scarring of the liver and the dietician struggles to get the nutrition status improved as patient has not been eating normal diet for prolonged period. They all do fantastic job. What medicine is poor at doing, is understanding the patient's wish that she has decided that her life is coming to an end, she has no intention to fight her alcohol dependence which is the root cause of all her medical conditions. We seldom have a chance to look further, what is the cause for the alcohol dependence. The blood tests and scans do not show the results of that!

Finally, there is a measure of collusion between society and medicine, orchestrated via the media's unrealistic and unbalanced portrayal of medical progress and success. Politicians promise of cure of dementia in next generation, and charities promise fight out cancer in next decade. Expectations of continuing therapeutic options delay the inevitable conversations crucial in developing a mutual understanding of how dying should occur. Despite important progress, cultural forces affecting both patients and doctors continue to prevent us from talking openly about the end of our lives.

Is dying becoming lonely, mechanical and dehumanised? Probably increasingly yes. Most deaths occurring in intensive care units occur in the end based on numbers derived from machines and graphs on the screen. It is also paradoxical, in the richest country in the world, USA, and in the poorest countries, poor people manage to die with dignity. Either they are uninsured or can't afford the medical takeover of their death.

MANNERS OF DEATH

Human life is a biological process. The internal environment of the body is constantly maintained by the physiologic processes termed as homeostasis. For convenience of study we divide these processes based on the functionality and organs, such as respiratory system (breathing and oxygenation) the cardiovascular system (heart and blood flow) digestive system (energy and nutrition). Then there are balance mechanisms of fluid, acidity, enzymes, ions and cells. The nervous system controls the regulation, includes brain and numerous chemical secretions like hormones. Any derangement of singular or multiple elements can be root cause of death, no wonder we die! It is astonishing that we live! All these systems can be affected by disease process or gradual age related and other changes. Of course, there is external threat of infection, trauma and poison toxicity.

The four manners of death are the four main categories in which death can occur that a pathologist will look for when he or she is examining the deceased. Natural Causes, quite simply when the body ceases to function of its own accord or if there are mitigating medical factors such as terminal illness, cardiac arrest or respiratory failure, which would bring about death - this is generally referred to as death by natural causes. Homicide, the taking of one human life by another human being by means of pre-meditated murder. The term premeditated means to have purposely planned. Accidental Death, as the term would suggest the death of an individual by means of an unexpected event. Suicide, the deliberate taking of one's own life due to extreme emotional distress often brought about by severe depression. Suicide is neither accidental nor is it classified as death by misadventure simply because the individual has set about on a course of action that would end with their own inevitable death.

WHERE YOU WANT TO DIE

" A man should die in his hut, lying in his bed, with his brothers and sons around him to hear his last words; he should die with his mind still alert and should be able to speak clearly even if only softly; he should die peacefully and with dignity, without bodily discomfort or disturbance; he should die loved and respected by his family". (Middleton, on Lugbara death in Uganda, in "Death and the regeneration of life")

In contemporary society, all over the world there are few choices for an anticipated planned death. They include, own home, acute care hospital ward, intensive care, a hospice, and a residential or nursing care home. Sudden deaths in natural setting, like on trekking or at sea on a cruise, as long as person was in readiness, can also be seen as good deaths. These were deaths, where dying is spared the stress and anxiety of the long dying trajectory. Each place has its own charm and it is for you to make the choice.

My grandmother had only one wish about her dying, she did not want to die in any medical facility. She almost told every person in the family, almost beggingly not to "put her in the hospital" at end of her life. Dying in your own home has the benefit of familiarity of the surrounding. There is no protocol to get adjusted to. There are down sides. First, medical input like pain control may be compromised. In United Kingdom NHS offers excellent nursing care service for home palliative care. This may not be universally available in many countries. Second, the way you will be remembered by your family may change due to your dying at home. You may not to wish your end of life state to be shared with your family. My grandmother died peacefully at home. I was not present at the time. It is often you remember the person, in context to the last interaction you had with them, and one may hope it is not the death bed.

Dying in intensive care or in an acute care hospital bed is highly medicalised. You are likely to be under medical surveillance in the form of word rounds, blood tests, imaging reports. I am familiar with this form. There never is a true acceptance that patient is going to die until a decision is made to transfer the patient to a hospice. In true sense, in spite of all the training of dignity and end of life pathways existing in acute care settings, we are not best prepared to facilitate a good death. And to be fair to the setting, the objective of the critical care team is not to facilitate a good death.

Hospice and palliative care setting are more suited for facilitating end of life. Hospice is typically an option for patients whose life expectancy is six months or less, and involves palliative care (pain and symptom relief) to enable your loved one to live their final days with the high quality of life possible. Hospice care can be provided onsite at some hospitals, nursing homes, and other health care facilities, although in most cases hospice is provided in the patient's own home. With the support of hospice staff, family and loved ones are able to focus more fully on enjoying the time remaining with the patient. When hospice care is provided at home, a family member acts as the primary caregiver, supervised by the patient's doctor and hospice medical staff. The hospice team makes regular visits to assess your loved one and provide additional care and services, such as speech and physical therapy or to help with bathing and other personal care needs.

As well as having staff on-call 24 hours a day, seven days a week, a hospice team provides emotional and spiritual support according to the wishes and beliefs of the patient. They also offer emotional support to the patient's family, caregivers, and loved ones, including grief counselling. Palliative care and hospice movement has increasingly become popular part of the care profession inventory. Palliative care settings offer expanded role beyond medical set ups. Therapy may be able to deliver many aspects of Patient Dignity Inventory, mostly used in North American palliative care physicians. These include attending to symptom distress (pain, anxiety, depression) existential distress (way you look, your job roles) dependency (ability to perform simple tasks) peace of mind (concerns about spiritual life, unfinished business) and social support (help from friend and family). Some residential care homes can provide combined experience of dying at familiar surroundings, as well as expertise in providing palliative care to the dying.

DRIVE TOWARDS DEATH

Most deaths occur as a natural phenomenon. There is increasing trend in society to control of the events. Quite correctly so. There is classic syringe driver induced oblivion to the switching off of the respiratory support. Voluntary acts of refusal to eat and drink, refusal for therapeutic fluid administration to accelerate death have been requested. Of course, the issues of suicide, assisted death and euthanasia have been much publicised and debated. There are many other ways people who have taken control of their destiny.

The concurrent or mutually opposing action" of the two fundamental drives, Eros and Thanatos, are supposed to explain "the phenomena of life". With Eros as the God of love and

Thanatos as the God of death, synonymous with the so-called death drive, we might even feel a hint of romanticism.

Thanatos v/s Eros

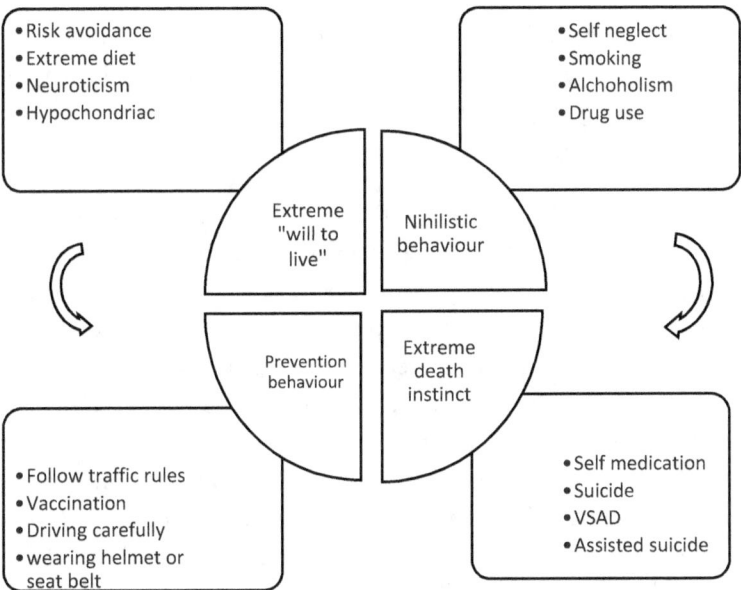

Illustration2. Extreme attitudes towards death on long term and short term.

EROS, representing the confluence of all those tendencies within us that aim to preserve life, and Thanatos, representing the impulse toward death, are central forces in human existence. Eros (the will to live) and Thanatos (death instinct) have been major themes of artists within the western tradition. The reasons for contemporary attitudes toward death are complex; the widespread abandonment in the twentieth century of traditional religious beliefs, found in Christian, Hindu, Buddhist and Judaic notions, entertaining the possibility of life's continuation after death through resurrection, reincarnation, or memory is one. Hope for the eventual triumph over death by means of continuing progress in medical technology is another. The loss of appropriate cultural rituals and symbols to express the meaning of death and to memorialize the dead in the context of life is also a factor. Finally, the literal banishment and isolation of the dying from the living in medical encampments effectively removes dying from public visibility.

THANATOS is known as the "death drive". Freud believed that human beings have an unconscious desire to destroy both themselves and others. Thanatos is believed to be an extension of the Freudian theory of the pleasure drive. Freud believed that the goal of human existence was to appease the pleasure principle, and Thanatos derives pleasure out of destruction. Freud described Thanatos as the process of returning to the inorganic, making that which is wholesome living and beautiful, dead, decrepit, and utterly destroyed. It is also known that when exposed to continued thought of death people show subtle nihilistic changes like smoking and excessive eating. It would be interesting to see sales figures from sugar and confectionery industry during the time of virus pandemic.

The idea that humans have an innate drive towards death and destruction is not a new idea and can be seen in various forms throughout history. Death has often been characterized by the colour black in classical symbolism, and can be seen as the darker half to the Yin Yang and even used for names of horrible diseases such as the Black Death. As for the idea that humans have a certain love for death and destruction, it is not hard to see how Sigmund Freud could have come up with this theory.

Eros is the drive to live and create. Freud was not the first philosopher to contemplate the ideas of Eros, lust, and love. Once again going back to the ancient Greeks, Plato philosophized that Eros had two dimensions where we love not only by carnal and lustful attractions, but also an internal love that goes beyond mere physical attraction. Even the phrase "platonic love", a love that is chaste and non-sexual comes from Plato's philosophy on Eros believing that love does not necessarily have to be physical.

Freud does not speak of Thanatos in substantive terms, he was wary of it and did not see it as having its own energy. Eros (love) takes the death drive into itself and renders it invisible. The death drive is a return to life's purest form. Freud introduced the concept of the death drive as a negative concept in opposition to the drive for life. So, whilst Eros is paired with the energy of 'libido', Thanatos has no such equivalent energy.

NON FUI, FUI, NON-SUM, NON CURO

The stoic view, one that does not incite despair or fear but instead inspires an acceptance of the universe, our fate and our eternal place in the living reality. Ancient Romans had the words inscribed on their funeral monuments. They may be translated as "I was not, I was, I am not, I care not". This epitaph is attributed to Epicurus, a Greek born philosopher of 4th century BC. Epicurus was attempting to rid the mankind of the fear of death which arises from certain religious beliefs. At that time religions believed that those violating particular standards will suffer eternal torment.

We did not exist before we were born, and so had no cares then.

We recall nothing before we were born. So why worry about not existing after death? You dint worry about not existing for millions of years before birth. It seems odd to even think of ourselves as entities which existed before our birth or will after our death. If indeed nothing awaits us after death, it is clear that we would not care about anything at all. The implied assertion, if it is not expressly stated, is that we have only one life and it should be lived as pleasantly as possible.

Since the advent of modern religions, tendency is to express hope in a residing in vaguely described heaven and contemplate with God. Perhaps the cessation of their lives did not disturb the ancients as it seems to disturb us today. It has seemed to disturb us for quite some time, especially since the belief in religion has become difficult to maintain. Modern materialism and individualism have glorified the self, and that would seem to make the belief that the self will vanish rather difficult to accept.

SUMMARY

Society and law, needs to change to allow patients a dignified death of their choice. Terminally ill patients should be allowed to choose how their death should occur. Patients should have the right, as a last rite to have water from Ganges, prayer to almighty, cuddle from a family member or sedative hypnotic syringe driver to induce oblivion.

COVID ON MY WARD

Like the falling man from the World trade building,

The boy in Tiananmen square without any shielding,

Like a moth rushing towards the flame with disregard,

I was sitting looking at my specialist ward,

Asking myself, are you willing and capable? Or unwilling capable?

May be, you are willing incapable, Or perhaps unwilling incapable.

I am mere mortal, don't know a thing,

I asked God, what he would do, be as a being.

I will walk on the ward where fellow men lie in bed,

Willing and capable? will try and help out instead,

I am not lured by the after-life reward,

awaiting answers, why there is COVID on my ward?

4 INFLUENCE OF RELIGION

No one owns religion. Religion owns concept of supernatural, including God. Humans, people, own religion, because religions were invented by us. So, we have the right to change it, continuously, as we learn more and understand our life better. We all know Santa is not real. In presence of currant scientific knowledge, no intelligent person can believe in supernatural superstitions. I refer to **Augusto Compte**'s vision for an evolution of religion alongside science, just like any other stream of knowledge. This is not a debate about whether there is a God or not. In the same premise of scientific knowledge, unlike religions, modern society gives humans the freedom in making their own choice about personal beliefs.

LEARNING FROM RELIGION

Religions have been here for a very long time. They have absorbed all the best and beautiful things, what works to keep the human society running. Just because we can conclusively reject supernatural powers, we don't need to discard religion as a basis of our society. It has its charm. Humans beings face painful events in life including loss of loved one and loss of our own life. Religions have understood and managed the processes very well. There has to be a process to subscribe to these clever ways without succumbing to the superstitious beliefs. Most useful and attractive ideas of all religions must be retained in a society.

Religions have been clever to absorb and transfer nonreligious events over centuries and benefit from their wisdom. Hinduism adapted festival of light into Diwali, celebration of colours into Holi and marking of solstice into Sankranti. Christianity too, converted pagan winter festival as Christmas and Islam converted most majestic temples into mosques when their rulers occupied India. As a first step of embracing best and beautiful aspects of religion, one should embrace all religions without their impractical elements. Then we can choose the elements. Like we can learn about compassion and mindfulness from Buddhism and ignore reincarnation and bardo concepts.

Religion based society promotes acceptance of morality, though it is defined by the scripture. If that scripture requires you to declare a crusade or jihad, you have an obligation to shun it. Religious activities improve spirit of community and promote good living. They also encourage gratitude and charitable giving. Religions recognised deep rooted selfish and competitive human behaviour and over time managed it using various beliefs. Whereas the concept of afterlife, punishment and reward after death can't be practiced, the need for managing these human qualities remain relevant. Without this approach, the secular society will be deprived of the colours, vibrance, melody and grandeur of religion inspired activities.

Approaching end of life and events after death are very stressful for everyone concerned. Need for support from community and family are at its peak. Religion helps to rally around the mourner help them express grief, at the same time give a structure towards a definitive period of mourning and encourage them to return to normal life. The rituals involved are symbolic and compensate for the grief and help to make the transition. Religions are wise, not to expect us to deal with the emotions of our own. Religions largely help to prepare the person towards death awareness, by loosening the grip of the ego on life. I have discussed concept of sannyasa in Hinduism.

RELIGIOUS EXPLOITATION OF DEATH

Exploitation of people who are vulnerable, helpless and lost control in trying to help a dying person has occurred over and again for thousands of years. As soon as our forebrain was big enough to be able to imagine a nonphysical entity, religion and gods were born. The pyramidal hierarchy of social system needed both fearful and influential powers to control mass public. There was no better subject than end of life, for such purpose. People were helpless due to impending loss of the dear ones but also did not understand the phenomena of death at all. Imaginations ran havoc. Concept of afterlife, hell and heaven, good and bad deeds which can influence your life after death, fear of god were all invented. The concepts were augmented by good and bad gods who could reward or punish you for your deeds. Few people who had the powers on their side made the rules of social system. They could influence everyone and those who did not obey the rules could be punished with the help of the believers.

This process of fear and anxiety related to unknow around death, dead and the aftermath of death, has repeated in so many generations, and for such long time, it is now difficult talk anything different about it. It will perhaps take some generations to assimilate our knowledge of science, medicine, psychology, human thinking and technological advancement to defeat deep entrenched attitudes and belief regarding end of human life. Religion deals with the problem of death by providing a belief system that denies the very notion of death, via the promise of an afterlife. However, due to the complexity of human cultures, different modes of religious beliefs and psycho-social differences, reliability of the religion and attitude towards death, cannot solely explain issues of the individual belief towards death and dying. If religion gives a blanket of comfort, a solace and some relief form anxiety, in the difficult moment of life, it is very welcome. However, it should not come with pretense of hope of afterlife, incarnation and other misguided beliefs to blind faith. That is burying your head in sand. Nothing could be far from the truth.

Isha had not slept all night thinking of her friend. Her friend has been unwell for some time and in pain. The illness was getting worse day by day. Isha had seen people dying before and feared the same may happen to her friend. She was prepared to do anything to stop this. Anything. But in the medieval era, where she lived, nothing she could think which would help her friend. She had heard of a group of wizards in the neighboring village who had power to communicate with a supreme entity. They could solve problem, any problem. So, she decided to visit them and ask for help.

The wizards had this problem before. Near and dear people of someone about to die would come and visit them and ask for help. They were in business of selling supreme power and would use anything they can think of, to make the prophecy believable. Of course, they were aware that neither them nor the supreme power had any influence on human disease or suffering. But hey wanted to influence and control the mass. Also perhaps reassure people, make them less disappointed, less angry and give some hope.

Wizards gave Isha knowledge of prayer and explained how it would reduce pain and suffering of her friend. Isha would accept any suggestion, any straw of hope. She just wanted to do something to help. The prayers carried on, friend was getting weaker and frail. But in her mind Isha felt relief that there was something she could do. A sense of control that not everything was lost. But one day her friend died. She was hurt, disappointed, angry and went to the wizards. They had expected this.

Wizard explained to Isha that her friend had not actually died. Just her spirit had left her body for now. The spirit needed some help to find a right path to either integrate with the supreme power or be reborn inside another body. Not all is lost. Not all is lost, Isha felt better and decided to follow the instructions of the wizard to help her friend's spirit. They helped her to dispose the physical remains of her friend in an appropriate way which could be approved by the supreme power. Everyone was a winner. The spirit found the right place for resting, or so was told by the wizard. Wizard now has a lifelong believer in supreme power, who would do anything to please the wizard. And Isha lived in hope that she did something to help her friend and has learnt a new way of life, which would help her soul when she died.

Let us look at death in a very selfish way. Everything you do, every action has a reaction, a consequence, and you need to deal with it. You are responsible for the effects of your action and normally you will be there to face it. Dying is the only action, you will not be able to deal with the consequences, as you will not be there. Someone else has to step in your shoes, but guaranteed it will not be you. You help everyone to do it, and I have discussed some practical measures, but you will not be responsible for your death or the aftermath of it. A recognition of our own mortality can, ironically, trigger nihilistic behaviors like smoking, drinking and overeating.

Not all religions and cultures accept death as a natural inevitable end of human life. Like politics, root of success of religion is its very character of deceptive ambiguity. And exploiting that ambiguity of end of life, religion is at its best. Death is depicted as a result of sin, or unacceptable deeds according to the scriptures of the particular sect. For some it could be eating beef, polygamy, gambling, consuming alcohol or even not undergoing prescribed religious ceremony could be that sin. Looking at this perspective, death could be scary. If you think you were made by god to live forever, then obviously you will be worried about the mortal nature of life.

THE CONCEPT OF SOUL

Many religions teach that soul or spirit or atma gives the body biological energy. Upon death the body decays and spirit are liberated. What happens to your spirit after your death is described in various religious texts. There is also encouragement to distinguish between material life and spiritual life, and how the material life will end with death and spiritual life will continue. Even suggestion that your soul will elevated to a higher level if you have led a highly spiritual life. There is nothing wrong in practicing what you believe. But surely, a life fulfilled with sense duty, humanity, compassion, care, helping everyone around you as best as you can be equally worthy of living, spiritual or not. You can certainly live a good life, nonmaterialistic life without being overtly spiritualistic.

Description of the soul, life, jeeva or atma, weather it is mortal or immortal always accompanied by questions if soul is material or immaterial? As the body is made of nothing but atoms and known physical processes of nature, soul can't be outside this physical entity. So, it can't be immaterial. And even if there is a physical soul, it can't exist or escape after death. People think about an immaterial soul that persists after the death. They have in mind some sort of blob of spirit energy that takes up residence near our body. If they refer to biological process of life, the biochemical activity, the flow of energy in homeostasis, surely such energy comes to termination, on cessation of chemical processes producing energy.

In mythical stories, there is descriptions of physical soul. Lord Shiva gave his soul to a disciple who was carrying it in southern India. The divine forces tricked the disciple, Ravana, to keep the soul on the ground, and the soul became inseparable from earth.

I have physically touched this soul in the Shiva temple in Gokarna, in southern India.

The Modern English word soul, is derived from old English word sáwel. The original concept behind the word mean "coming from or belonging to the sea or lake", because of the Germanic and pre-Celtic belief in souls emerging from and returning to sacred lakes. The Koine Greek word life, spirit, consciousness, is derived from a verb meaning "to cool, to blow", and hence refers to the breath. Atman is a Sanskrit word that means inner self or soul. In Hinduism, a jiva or jeev, is a living being, or any entity imbued with a life force. The Quran, the holy book of Islam, distinguishes between the immortal Ruh (spirit) and the mortal Nafs (self, soul). The immortal Ruḥ, drives the mortal Nafs, which comprises temporal desires and perceptions necessary for living.

TALKING ABOUT DEATH

Irrespective of the fact that death related experience is terrifying and affects individual perception of the phenomenon, open and objective discussion about it can still help the individuals with anxiety problem to cope. Awareness about the end of life is such a powerful emotion, it will require an encouragement from the society and people around to calm the individual and to inspire them to see death as normal and inevitable.

When we do get around to thinking about death, it is with a sense of fear, panic or denial. It is time to adopt a more modern and enlightened view of death, without suspicion or fear, but understanding the reality of it and giving some thought to it throughout life, so that death is one of many areas of perspective that inform the way we live. Western societies avoid talking about death, because we have lost faith in transcendent life.

It's not only relatives and friends who might find it difficult to talk about what's happening. The dying themselves often find it very hard to express what they are feeling or what they would like. Talking about death is not easy thing to do. There is always fear that you may say something wrong or upset someone. There is also sense of fear of loss as the topic you are talking about, you don't understand well. You are not sure that how much truth about impending death has been discussed with the person dying or the relatives. There is always risk that others may be pretending everything is alright. Some relative disagree to take part in the conversation, and may expect the professionals to talk about death and prefer not to engage.

Fear of own mortality prevents people from talking about death. Often person is in denial about death or is frustrated and angry about what is happening to him. Talking about death may make things worse in these situations. The ability or willingness of someone dying to talk about their own death may be affected by similar factors. Lack of privacy in acute care hospitals is major factor in not being able to start the conversation about death. Dying person may choose to talk to a professional person like a doctor, nurse or a lawyer and not a relative. Some older people may not have close friends or surviving relatives they wish to speak. Talking about death usually brings about a lot of feelings, anxiety, fear, sadness and awkwardness. As a culture, we tend to pretend it does not happen. But when it happens, strong emotions come up, So, it is incredibly important for all generations to talk about death, ahead of time, so that feelings can be faced, processed and relationships set straight.

FEAR AND ANXIETY

There are two types of fears. One, innate, inborn fear, probably deep seated in our neural system, honed by millennia of evolutionary experience, a protective or survival reflex of instinct. The other is acquired, more learned through observation or experience, seated in in the most advanced, creative and imaginary part of the brain. Both these types of fears can cause fear of death and anxiety. The innate part of fear of death is about extinction, being no more, sense of end and inevitability. The innate fear of loss affects at all ages, impermanence of objects in childhood to fear of losing the tooth, all are innate fears. The acquired fear of death is more imaginary. It is through observation of behaviour of other people, developed by cultural influence and can be conditioned. Perhaps fear of dentist or fear of losing your loved one are examples of acquired fears.

We can't eradicate the fear, if the cause of the fear is unknown. And we can't make inquiry into death unless we eradicate the fear of death. Unless you make your own fearless unbiased inquiry into something, you can't understand or embrace it. So, to understand death we need to address the fear of it, both innate and acquired. As long as death remains unknown, the fear gets compounded as the fear of the unknow. So, the circle has to be broken somewhere. In the last chapter I have discussed how innate fears can be addressed, by simply bringing them to the conscious level, simply by talking or reading about it.

"The idea of death, the fear of it, haunts the human animal like nothing else," wrote Earnest Becker in his book, The Denial of Death. It is the innate fear which motivates us to many things. People often fear dying in pain. They don't want to be there when it happens. However, if and when death is inevitable, but likely to come easily, all the evidence suggests that people generally take it remarkably calmly. Some theorists say, but the lack of overt fear is due to some form of denial. The causes of fear are complex, thanatophobia (and our fear of death in general) can arise from many factors. Fearing a sudden or prolonged death, fearing a painful or gruesome death, fearing the unknown or "What lies beyond?", fearing for the well-being of loved ones/survivors in the future, and fears rooted in past painful or negative life experiences.

Two-way process of interaction between religion and fear is the dominant source of anxiety. Religion on one hand, is supposed to protect us from fears and all evil. Religious people do most life activities to abide by the rules of religion so that they are spared of bad things. Unfortunately, religion also has profound influence on way people feel about what happens to them after their death. The concept of heaven and hell, rebirth, judgement day recompense, and all stories in scriptures can induce fear and anxiety. We need to become death aware and stop believing in superstitious beliefs during course of our life to overcome these fears.

Spinoza described that humans are able to overcome problem of death. From Spinoza's point of view, death is only a relative evil, namely in the relation to our nature. "Death can play the role of evil only for men who lack the higher forms of understanding. A sensuous man who is dragged by his passions and imaginations, passive being who is not able of really act, for such a man, death is the absolute evil". Such is afraid of death and is unable to save himself from dealing continuously with the painful idea of death. Instead of living his life in its fulness, he steadily suffers said Spinoza.

Pinnacle of Life

	Negative thinking	**Mental ability**	Positive thinking	
	Self obsession	Self awareness	Selfless identity	
Death anxiety	Worry about possible things (future)	Ability to identify future	Successful life plan	**Death awareness**
	Focus on loss and worry	Ability to identify threats	Gratitude	
		Attitude		

Chart 3. How mental attitude and ability can affect development of death awareness or death anxiety.

As human capacity of thinking improved, thought process regarding self, ability to think about future and ability to imagine and therefore predict risks has developed. Self-awareness is powerful and can be both constructive and opposite. Self-awareness allows you to develop a selfless identity, thereby giving pleasure in giving and positive outlook towards detachment and death awareness. On negative side, excess focus on self can cause death anxiety due to inability to develop detachment. Humans have ability to think about their own thoughts and therefore can think about future. People with positive thought processes can use the ability to identify future for life planning. But looking at future can also create mortality awareness and anxiety. I have discussed some issues about coping with the anxiety in the final chapter.

CONCEPT OF HEAVEN

Processing a horrific experience like the loss of a loved one using rationality and logic does help when you're trying to make sense of things, but not as much during those times you're feeling helpless and emotionally vulnerable. I can see how believing in God can help there.

That said, what do believers do with this God? Do they rage at him for cruelly taking their parent, spouse, or child away from them? Or do they surrender to their helplessness, thanking him for putting their loved ones "in a better place", begging him to reunite them one day?

Jack fell down, broke his crown and was serious. Jack was a good bloke, middle of the road. In fact, he was so average that friends used to call him fifty-fifty. When he was taken to intensive care unit fate played a trick on him, fifty-fifty. His body was on ventilator support but his spirit had escaped and made its way to another world. Jack wondered in this new world and found many strange places. He came to the main gate where the man in charge of the judgment again appeared confused. He said "mate you are fifty-fifty, would you like to go to heaven or hell?" Jack dint know much about afterlife, but he had heard about hell in his religious education class. He remembered in time, that hell is an afterlife location for eternal punishment. He chose to go to heaven.

Walking down the main street he found many buildings servicing heavenly activities for the subscribers of various scriptures. Valhalla, where Nordic strongmen gathered to drink beer all day, preparing for the next fight. There was thirteen layers heaven made out of Cipactli's head housing the Aztec warriors. Jannah, the garden paradise, luminescent, white and in the clouds was busy with Islamic believers. He also saw the court of king Indra, with dancing apsaras where he could smell aroma of heavenly curry. Then there were Tian, the Garden of Eden, Vyraj, and others. Jack was, fifty-fifty, kind of atheist, nonsubscriber. He could have walked into any building.

Jack was given room in the magnificent palace, the land of milk and honey. There were nymphs singing, angels dancing and beautiful eyed virgins giving him company. Jack settled down and suddenly remembered his life on beautiful planet. Being fifty-fifty, he still had some characters from earthly life, the "sense of time". It is a very important concept for the mortals. Jack was not too impressed by the menu, he was more of a vindaloo kind of bloke, and milk honey and dates were not his taste. But he was attracted to a blue-eyed virgin. How long can I stay here? he asked. She was a bit confused, "forever" was the reply.

Jack was troubled by two chains of thoughts. First, he thought no logic, to the concept of the company of the pure. If I have intimate relationship with the company, then, there won't be any virgins, I will have human life, the family, children etc. all over again. Potentially that could even become a hell on heaven (as opposed to hell on earth) he thought. That is not the way to live, he decided. But then what good is the company, same over and again, for as long as you can think, even hundreds of years. Even in the company of the blue-eyed virgin, the land of milk and honey, forever and forever, would be dull, boring and tedious, he thought. There was no sense of time, no emotions, surprises, loss or win, good or bad, nothing at all. The loss of sense of time had taken everything away. Jack was not quite ready, just in case he met the God or any one higher up. Should I thank him for putting me up in this better place, or should I be very angry, because he has taken me away from my earthly life. More he thought about it, more he was getting confused, he needed more time.

Jack politely said good bye to all company in the heaven, thanked the bloke at the gate for letting him in and decided to make his way back to his mortal *body. His body woke up with feeling, someone has been breaking his ribs. The intensive care staff were overjoyed to have done a successful CPR.*

It was all a dream. Jack woke up from the dream, he was still disturbed by the thought of death, and what to do, if he really died. He went to see his friend, a minister and guru. He reassured Jack, asked him to live a good life, here and now, middle of the road, and not to worry about things after life. Jack lived happily ever after.

Religion is the only concept that has lived on for millennia without being adapted to the advances in human society! So, what makes religion eternal and everlasting? How can anything possibly have such a strong grasp on humanity for millennia? By playing on humanity's worst fears — mortality — religion thrives as a crucial tool to bring peace and tranquility. By extension, we then tend to turn to prayers for any of life's uncertainties that come our way!

There may have been a point in time when using fear of God as way to bring order, civility and even healthy living made sense. But at the moment, the impact of religion on humanity is catastrophic! The abuse of religion is now singlehandedly responsible for causing massive rifts among people and heinous crimes! While the original goals of religion may have been noble, we have used religion to construct certain walls around us. In the name of religion, we wash our sins by surrendering them to an invisible power, thereby continuing the cycle of sinning and claiming redemption.

We have moved forward in most other dimensions of life. We use modern medicine. We use modern food techniques. We use modern modes of communication. Yet, *in the dimension of religion, we haven't evolved at all!*

Now more than ever, it is so important for humanity to come together and set aside differences.

AFTERLIFE

Universal belief is powerful. We all believe in money. In reality there is no such thing. Because we universally believe, honour and value the quantum attached to money, its existence is possible. Similar argument can be made towards universal beliefs without evidence of existence, such as afterlife, heaven and religion itself. We need to question the utility of these beliefs to the human life and society. According to Islamic scholars, life is a test that ends with death: "*Every soul shall have a taste of death and we test you by evil and by good by way of trial.*" (Quran). Christianity shares this judgment day vision as well. Christianity and Islam are "other world" explanations for death. There are many of these kinds of religions. Norse mythology granted those who died well in combat an afterlife in Valhalla with Odin or in Freyja's field. In Greek mythology, the good passed to Elysian Fields. These otherworld explanations offer our lives as a transition from wherever we were before to a resting place beyond. Life after death does exist, just not for the person died!

Afterlife is a wishful thinking. It is hard to imagine *non-being*, and from this hardship, from wishful thinking, and from a sense of justice, we yearn for an afterlife. To make meaning of our lives we want this life to be part of a learning curve that doesn't just end, unfinished. Religion, and the afterlife, serve to make us think of death as less important and less of a barrier. We should not doubt the power of the idea that death is not final. It is not just a personal rejection of death that compels people towards religious ideas of an afterlife - scholar of religion William Sims

Bainbridge calls these *primary compensators*. The *secondary* type of reaction against death is social. People like having something comforting to tell others to lessen the gravity of death of a loved one, making the social dynamics less morbid and more positive in outlook. Hence, there are a range of subtle internal psychological factors that give us a need and a want for an afterlife and/or for a purpose of death that transcends life and mitigates the disaster of losing a human being forever.

To manage that fear we long ago developed replacement, more positive abstract thoughts such as eternal life, salvation, liberation, and reincarnation; and we developed religions and spiritualities to manage those ideas.

CONCEPT OF HELL AND PUNISHMENT

Belief in an old-fashioned, everlasting Hell hasn't gone away. But Hell has long been assailed as one of religions cruder means of maintaining control.

The ancient Jews had no concept of 'heaven' as a place of rewards, or 'hell' as a place of punishment, but instead held that all humans went to a shadowy and monotonous afterlife after death: Sheol. Rewards and punishments accrued to people in this life, not in the life to come. Similarly, the ancient Greeks believed that everyone went to the lethargic and gloomy underworld of Hades. Over time, the Catholic Church warmed to the idea that purgatory was an actual place, akin to heaven and hell. Just as the bifurcation of the afterlife seemed to offer more moral nuance than a single shadowy underworld where everyone ended up, so the emergence of purgatory seemed to offer more moral gradation than the stark either/or of heaven and hell. By the time of the Protestant Reformation, most people assumed that they would end up in purgatory after death, since few were good enough for immediate entry to heaven or bad enough for automatic consignment to hell.

Naraka is the Hindu equivalent of Hell, similar to Jahannam in Islam, where sinners are tormented after death. Naraka is also the abode of Yama, the god of Death. It is described as located in the south of the universe and beneath the earth. Because of the strong images the narratives of hell contain, they are excellent means to catch the attention of the audience. The social function of hell is to protect the social order, the security of the people and specially to protect the privileges of those on top of the hierarchy. Since gifts to the priests are matched with specific punishments in hell that they release from, one economic function of hell seems to be as a source of income for the priests.

Not all aspects of religion advocate fearful notion of death. Buddha's first noble truth is prescription for preparation towards death. "Life is filled with pain and grief because human desire for death not to occur. Dukkha (suffering and frustration or grief) comes from difficulty in facing basic facts of life, that everything is transitory. Suffering arises from clinging to impermanent things.". Further in the fourth truth, he described eight-fold path or steps for individual development. Death as means of contemplation of impermanence. The step are right kind of view, thought, speech, action, livelihood, mindfulness, effort and concentration. Taoism considers death is part of a natural change. No man's explanation of life is absolute. There is no life without death.

DEATH AS PRODUCT OF SIN

In our subconscious mind, it is not possible for us to accept or imagine that our existence will come to an end, by a natural cause. We think it can only happen by an evil act or a bad cause. Hence there is always fear, retribution, punishment and sin from bad acts associated with it. This concept is probably the most contributory factor towards death anxiety. A clear division, either one is assured of eternal life with divine powers or doomed to punishment and hell, can be source of fear for those who believe in the scriptures. Concept of judgement day, and belief that we are just travelers who are passing through this life before reaching other life does not give much comfort.

The story of Genesis tells us about the original sin of mankind which results in mortality becoming essential. Milton retells the story in "Paradise Lost" by personifying Sin. Book describes Sin as daughter of Satan and mother of Death. By implication, sin resulted in mortality of humans, and often the original sin is referred to be influenced by the serpent. In Hebrew the root word for Eve (Hawa) means breath, living can also mean a snake. Mythologically snakes are symbol for fertility, change and immortality. This widely held belief of sin, evil and relation to death has made it difficult to accept a normal death. In every death people look for a dark side, a sin or punishable offence. After all our existence is influenced by the original sin, and we are children of serpent's influence. Both extremes, largely post religious west, and blindly faithful other parts of the world, issue of death still remains enigmatic to the general public.

SUMMARY

Religion gives solace and comfort at the time of distress. But it can evoke false hopes. There is a lot we can learn from religion. The belief also provides concepts which needs to be scrutinised. Some religions value and respect life, and treat life as sacred. This can have influence in preventing nihilistic attitude.

Pinnacle of Life

ELEMENTS

My elements need to go back, to where they came from,

It's not my soul, but my body, need to complete the term.

To my mother earth, give me a place to rest,

Take back my weight, you have been bearing all my life,

To the moon, star and everlasting sun,

Take my energy, you have been giving to me all my life,

To the wind, fresh air and blow of breeze,

Take back my breath, I have been gasping you all my life,

To the burning fire, the heat and the blast,

Take back warmth of my heart, you have given me all my life,

To the water and salt, the snow, rain and majestic sea,

Take my blood, the flow, you have circulated in me all my life,

To the celestial space and unseen world,

Take my thoughts, I have wondered in your yard all my life,

Thank you, father, choosing me to be born,

On this beautiful planet, but it is time to return.

5 MEMENTO MORI

REMEMBER YOU MUST DIE

Memento Mori is believed to have originated from an ancient Roman tradition. After a major military victory, the triumphant military generals were paraded through the streets to the roars of the masses. The ceremonial procession could span the course of a day with the military leader riding in a chariot drawn by four horses. There was not a more coveted honour. The general was idolized, viewed as divine by his troops and the public alike. But riding in the same chariot, standing just behind the worshipped general, was a slave. The slave's sole responsibility for the entirety of the procession was to whisper in the general's ear continuously, "Respice post te. Hominem te esse memento. Memento mori!" "Look behind. Remember thou art mortal. Remember you must die!" The slave served to remind the victor at the peak of glory, this god-like adoration would soon end, while the truth of his mortality remained.

The point of this reminder isn't to be morbid or promote fear, but to inspire, motivate and clarify. The idea has been central to art, philosophy, literature, architecture, and more throughout history.

"Let us prepare our minds as if we'd come to the very end of life. Let us postpone nothing. Let us balance life's books each day...The one who puts the finishing touches on their life each day is never short of time."

The Stoics used Memento Mori to invigorate life, and to create priority and meaning. They treated each day as a gift, and reminded themselves constantly to not waste any time in the day on the trivial and vain.

Michel de Montaigne, known for creating the essay as a literary genre and regarded as the Father of Modern Scepticism, wrote in an essay titled *"That to Study Philosophy is to Learn to Die"*, of the ancient Egyptian custom where celebratory feasts concluded with the raising of a skeleton to the chant, "Drink and be merry, for such shalt thou be when thou are dead." In the height of celebration, Egyptian custom was to set remembrance to the frailness and fleetingness of festival. Through the visual of the skeleton and the pronouncing of the chant, celebrators reeled in the jollity to acknowledge the moment would soon pass so not to take it for granted.

Steve Jobs famously said *"Remembering that I'll be dead soon is the most important tool I've ever encountered to help me make the big choices in life. Almost everything — all external expectations, all pride, all fear of embarrassment or failure — these things just fall away in the face of death, leaving only what is truly important. Remembering that you are going to die is the best way I know to avoid the trap of thinking you have something to lose. You are already naked. There is no reason not to follow your heart."*

Today, the typical person doesn't think about death at all because it's uncomfortable, sad or scary. Fortunately, we're no longer cavemen afraid that we're going to be eaten by a lion, or ancient Romans afraid we'll be murdered by a gladiator, or Medieval sires afraid we'll fall victim to plague. Unfortunately, however, as the world has gotten safer and better, we start to think that we're going to live forever and that things are always going to go exactly our way. The Stoics would say that death is what gives life meaning – it's the cap at the end that helps us make the most of the time we've been given.

DANSE MACABRE

The Late Middle Ages was a period of devastation. A catastrophic plague, the Black Death, devastated Europe, killing an estimated 25 million people, third of the population. Out of the grim horrors and fight for survival grew an art genre called Danse Macabre, meaning Dance of Death. Like plague, Danse Macabre illustrates the all-conquering power of death. Paintings include kings with peasants, young with old, to convey that death comes for everyone.

Life is fleeting so best to not waste it on meaningless goods and pleasures. That's the message behind vanitas art. Inspired by the first chapter of Ecclesiastes ("vanity of vanity, all is vanity"), Dutch Golden Age artists of the 17th century used still-life as moral instruction. Artists emphasized the emptiness and futility of earthly items. Skulls, candles, hourglasses, watches, rotting fruit, wilting flowers, and fraying books sat atop a table to remind viewers just how precious life is.

Plagues, wars, and massacres aside, people of the Regency and Victorian eras dealt too with some of the highest infant mortality rates in history. Without vaccines to control illness, mothers lost the life of their new born, and sometimes their own, at an alarming rate. Documentation started to be kept in a yearly Bill of Mortality. To say death was on the public's mind would perhaps be an understatement.

The haunting reality of life's uncertainty showed itself in many forms: art, literature, architecture, and a new trend, jewellery.

Memento Mori rings were worn by everyone from Queen Victoria to the impoverished. Skeletal bands and skulls wearing a crown reminded wearers that death is the master of all.

Most images of memento mori are more constrained, and less dramatic. They might include a skeleton, an hour glass, the wheel of time, an overturned glass, or a winged boy holding an inverted torch represented in the context of a still life or portrait composition. Memento mori images range from a panel-picture representing decay and purification with a grotesque human head resembling a modem Dracula figure, accompanied by an hour glass, and scales, representative of the fifteenth and sixteenth century tradition of horror inspired art designed to warn the rich and great of the vanity of wealth and earthly titles, to more polite and controlled reminders found in Dutch and other still life and portrait paintings particularly in the seventeenth century.

While Memento Mori has fallen from consciousness compared to its historical relevance, mortality motivation is practiced modern life is fueling successful entrepreneurs, artists, athletes, authors, among others.

Death reflection describes a cognitive state of death awareness, one in which individuals put their lives in context, contemplate their meaning and purpose, and review how others will look upon them after they have passed. Death reflection is processed psychologically in what is known as the "cool" or cognitive system, which is characterized by deliberate, analytical, rational reactions based on systematic processing that is subject to intentional control.

MARANASATI

Mindfulness of death is a central teaching in Buddhism. The meditative practice Maranasati, meaning "death awareness," is considered essential to better living. It brings recognition to the transitory nature of one's physical life, and stimulates the question of whether or not one is making the right use of their fragile and precious life. According to the Maranasati, a monk should reflect on the many possibilities which could bring death and then turn his thoughts to the mental qualities he has yet to abandon.

Maranasati is one of the "Four Thoughts," which turn the mind towards spiritual practice. One set of Tibetan Buddhist contemplations on death come from the eleventh century Buddhist scholar Atisha. He is said to have said to his students that if a person is unaware of death, their meditation will have little power.

Atisha's contemplations on death: Death is inevitable, Our life span is decreasing continuously, Death will come, whether or not we are prepared for it, Human life expectancy is uncertain, There are many causes of death, The human body is fragile and vulnerable, At the time of death, our material resources are not of use to us, Our loved ones cannot keep us from death and Our own body cannot help us at the time of our death. Other Tibetan Buddhist practices deal directly with the moment of death, preparing the meditator for entering and navigating the Bardo, the intermediate stage between life and death. This is the theme of the popular Great Liberation through hearing during the intermediate state (Tibetan book of the dead).

DEATH INSTINCT

Sigmund Freud, in his book "Beyond the pleasure principle" concluded that all driving forces of life (instincts) fall in two major categories, life instinct (Eros) and death instinct (Thanatos). Life instincts create the energy of living, Freud termed as libido. Life instinct deal with basic survival, pleasure and reproduction. He maintained that life instincts were opposed by the self-destructive death instincts, known as Thanatos.

The concept of the death instincts was initially described by Freud as "the goal of all life is death." He believed that people typically channel their death instincts outwards as aggression. He further proposed that the death instincts were an extension of that compulsion wherein all living organisms have an instinctive "pressure toward death" which contrast to the instinct to survive, procreate, and satisfy desires. He explained that there is an urge in organic life to restore an earlier state of things, the inorganic state from which life originally emerged. The death drive then manifested itself in the individual creature as a force "whose function is to assure that the organism shall follow its own path to death".

Personality and life-span developmental psychologists have offered a different perspective on death awareness. In his classic epigenetic theory of development, psychologist Erik Erikson proposed that people progress through eight psychological stages of life, each of which involves a developmental crisis. He dedicated the last two of his eight stages of life to issues related to death. He proposed that in the final stage of life people become increasingly aware of death, which leads to a crisis between ego integrity and despair. Those who overcome this crisis experience ego integrity, finding coherence and meaning in their lives and accepting death. Those who succumb to this crisis experience despair, continuing to fear and dread death. Erikson proposed that, before reaching this stage, in the penultimate stage of life, which occurs throughout middle adulthood, people grapple with the notion that their lives are finite. They undergo a midlife crisis between generativity and stagnation, contributing to the next generation versus ceasing to be a productive member of society. He proposed that people who prevail over this crisis become generative by performing socially valuable work and mentoring members of younger generations. People who fall victim to this crisis, however, become stagnant by withdrawing from socially valuable work and mentoring activities

WHY SHOULD WE DIE?

Evolution and nature have perfected over millions of years, over many thousands of life cycles, the event of death and birth. Perhaps death is a way of clearing out for the next and younger generation. As a person lives through life, the cells and genes become damaged and age changes cumulatively difficult for the body and nature to maintain. So, it is easier for the nature to replace the person with younger individual. The older you get, higher the risk for the body organs or cells to cause disfunction resulting in disease like dementia or cancer. Younger progeny will also have benefit of selecting the fittest genetic pool from the older. This model has its downside. Every time an individual dies a generation of skills, knowledge and training are lost and the new generations has to do it all again.

The young look forward. The old look back. What matters to us changes as we get older. The prospect of death informs these changes. The young have an intellectual understanding that death comes to us all, but their mortality has not become real to them. For the old, mortality starts to sink in.

The only death that really scares me is the death of those I love, far more than my own. This is not to say that I don't want to live as long as possible, so long as I can function in some way and not be an excessive burden.

Most animals seem to have hardly any conception of mortality: to them, a dead body is just another object, and the transition between life and death unremarkable. We, on the other hand, tend to treat those who have passed away as "beyond human", rather than "non-human" or even "ex-human". We have developed social behaviors around the treatment of the dead whose complexity far exceeds even our closest living relatives' cursory interest in their fallen comrades.

You could say that humans invented death – not the fact of it, of course, but its meaning as a life event imbued with cultural and psychological significance. But even after many millennia of cultural development, we don't seem to be sure exactly what it is we've invented. The more we try to pin down the precise nature of death, the more elusive it becomes; and the more elusive it becomes, the more debatable our definitions of it.

Most of us would wish for a peaceful death after a long and well-lived life. Of course, not all of us get our wish. For some, death comes sooner than we would like, and that's one reason to fear it. Only recently has it become commonplace for death to come later than we would like. Death can now be deferred by mechanical and medicinal means for days, weeks, months or years – and that brings with it fears of its own: of impotence, dependency and pain. Nothing in the way our societies are constructed is at all suited to this new situation.

COVID-19 PANDEMIC

At end of last millennium, world mad preparation for a largescale disruption to our life. It was called millennium bug. All kind of scenarios were discussed. Contingency plans were made. The bug did not arrive. 20 years later, a bug arrived from Wuhan province from China, travelled around the globe using humans as vectors. The result is a catastrophic change. The virus causing this disease COVID-19has potential to spread from human to human, and possibly from human to animals and other way.

COVID -19 deaths are somewhat different from many previously recorded catastrophic events. These happened all over the globe. Simultaneously. We knew many were going to die, graves were dug in preparation, but we dint know who were going to die. The pandemic gave notice to governments and local bodies, there will be carnage, but the virus did not give much time for the individual. The virulence of the bug was such that the medical teams, even with their infection control knowledge and protective equipment succumbed to the infection. That meant the relatives were unable or not allowed to be with the affected individual. Most deaths happened in isolation.

The admission rates were so rapid, some relatives did not even know where their relatives were being treated. Medical facilities were over run by the sheer volume and scale of the attack. This was no fiction. World was running out of simple mouth masks and gowns. In the most developed nation in the world, reports showed scared medical staff were wearing ski goggles and rubbish bin sacks to protect themselves. The intensive care doctors have to make decision, the most difficult in their career, whom to intubate and whom to let go.

The virus did not discriminate. There were celebrities, doctors, political authorities, people of all age religion and colour were on the line. Social isolation added new level of anxiety in the society. Medicine will learn its lessons. But for the moment, there is no cure, no known drug to make patient better, no known knowledge how to stop it from spreading. It is the test of time. We were unprepared, massively unprepared. The success of medicine over the past century gave us that arrogance, that we are humans, our world can't be conquered. I worked a hospital during the pandemic, I was part of the reaction humanity experienced, the scare helplessness, and desire to help and do our best. The worse the pandemic got, better was the human resolve to help each other.

Reaction to news of impeding death, or any bad news, was studied and described by Elisabeth Kübler-Ross. She gave us our first clinical insights into the somewhat universal process of how human beings react to such situations. She provided us with a listing and explanation of the five common stages, which are well known. They usually occur in a cluster. Pandemic was no different. Denial, Anger, Bargaining, Despair and Acceptance are the stage.

There was a denial in every level, governments did not introduce preventive lock down measures quickly enough. There was talk of riding it out and developing herd immunity. People were still leaving to go on holidays. Political leaders declared it as just a flu. Statistics were circulated that majority of us will be OK. Denial is the intellectual and emotional rejection of something that is clear and obvious. Denial caused the delay and contributed to the long-term lack of preparation.

Anger is an emotional reaction in dealing with a problem. It is a way out from dealing with a problem. Pandemic caused wide spread anger. Anger was expressed towards every possible source. People in Wuhan were angry that they have to live through most stringent lock down procedures, at the same time people outside were angry that china could have done more to prevent the spread of the disease to rest of the world. We are used to a civilisation where government can fix it all. We were angry that government was not doing enough. Blaming, being hostile, refusing to follow rules are all signs of anger response to the pandemic.

Bargaining occurs when denial breaks down and we start to acknowledge reality but we're not ready to give up the illusion that we still have control. Agreement to follow the lock down measure was a bargaining mode. Sooner you follow the advice, sooner it will be over. Basically, we try to compromise to find an easier, less painful way. Authorities tried to encourage bargaining by offering supportive financial packages. Again, the facts that used for denial, namely, most of us will be OK, only elderly are at risk, I do not have underlying illness etc. were used for a psychological bargaining shield.

Despair and depression occur when there is no more room for denial. The reports of increasing number of deaths, the difficulties in treating the large volume of patients and the knowledge about complete lack of specific medical treatment compounded the anxiety and fear. There was hopelessness about the economy, jobs and future of everything. For the families of those who were affected, there was not much time to react. Events unfolded very quickly.

Acceptance is a stage when we start dealing with an appropriate response. Acceptance in case of coronavirus disease was to play individual roles. That included staying home, follow advice, washing hands. The response in institutional level was to cancel flights, sports and entertainment events, making arrangement for financial support etc.

Can we be death aware and death prepared for situations like COVID 19. Probably no. But the pandemic largely dealt with mass scale and volume of cases. On an individual level it was still the same. Same death anxiety, same family reaction to bereavement and same grief reaction. Neither religion nor medicine and science were able to control wide spread anxiety about the pandemic.

INDIVIDUAL RESPONSE

Individual person reacts in similar way to news of shock, it may be a new diagnosis of terminal illness or worsening of a known condition, the reaction is same. As described by Dr Kubler-Ross, they follow sequence or cluster of denial and isolation, anger and grievance, bargaining, depression and despair and eventually some acceptance and hope. Denial and isolation are an abrupt response, and is a healthy way of confronting uncomfortable situation and helps get on with life. It allows the person to collect themselves from a state of shock. Maintaining denial is rare and the denial can occur sporadically. Anger is normal physiologic reaction. Anger is usually due to resentment and questioning of self "why me?" angry reaction is difficult to cope for family and medical staff. Anger can be expressed at random towards all people and process involved. Bargaining happens in mind. Bargaining is a process of postponing the inevitable, for a brief period. It is a stage of agreement. Depression and despair are caused by sense of loss. This may happen in many facets like dysfunction, disfigurement, loss of social life, financial burden and loss of job role. some depression is preparatory to the final demise. Taking into account the impending loss, the management is difficult. Reassurance is not meaningful. Preparatory depression is necessary to get readiness for separation from life. It will also help to overcome anxiety.

Acceptance is the beginning of the end of struggle. Patients always been advised re "fight" against the disease. Medicine has a large role to play in making it difficult for the patient to accept the inevitable. Acceptance of one's death is not cowardly giving up, that is what some doctors make you feel. Contemplating the impending end with void of emotions will allow you look at other aspects for your bucket list. There is always a sudden change in attitude of a dying patient, a glimmer of hope, some new medicine, technique or person may be able to solve the problem. This end stage hopefulness is due to inability of acceptance.

WHY COVID IS DIFFERENT

Type of death seen I this epidemic is nothing like our generation has seen. Even in sudden deaths occurring in war, there is a profiling of who may die. We know there is a war, we anticipate some of brave soldiers may die, both sides. Some innocent people will die due to civilian casualties, but we anticipate that in the war zone. I famine and floods, again geographical distribution is followed. With COVID, by definition of pandemic, it could affect anybody. There is no predictability. There are no weapons, just a virus. NO vaccine, no proven treatment. There is no cease fire or relief efforts. Front line medical staff fought like soldiers, and some sadly died, and many more were infected. Psychologically this type of mass event causing death awareness, was never played out in the media. Governments used every possible means at their disposal to curb the effect of mass casualties. The role of epidemiologist, was played out in public. And yet, denial, psychological reluctance that it could happen, caused delay in response in every country.

COVID has caused mass death awareness and preparedness in the community. In the past, mass casualty events like world war, plague have caused massive cultural shift in the way people think about their life. We need to wait until the storm to pass, assess the economic damages it has left behind, and then the cultural response will become obvious. Never before simple measure like social distancing was used as effective tool for saving lives. The degree of infectivity meant the relatives, friends or priest could not visit you to comfort you in your last hours. The system was run over by sheer number and speed. There were no good byes, that is different.

Could we apply the "pillars of wisdom" about deaths occurring from COVID. I have discussed the five pillars in the final chapter. Even though the sequence of how COVID affected us is different, largely I believe we could have applied them both collectively and to the individuals. When declared pandemic, there was explosion of media coverage of death awareness. Though some appeared in numbers and graphs, and was not making connection to the real human tragedy, everyone watched it, every day. Death, played out on media has extensive audience, that is our human nature, it is deep rooted in our psyche, we reflect on our mortality watching others. COVID also ruptured the closed bubble we live in modern society. Our attitudes towards fellow citizens has changed, hopefully this will last. Hopefully we appreciate better times, more, specially the relative safety net of health care.

Death preparedness is a longer-term issue. As a country, our contingency supplies were very low. This was particularly evident in Unite States and the UK. States which had additional capacity like Germany, at least in early stages managed the outbreak better. Political establishments will think harder about making better provisions for preparedness in their planning process. Last minute hurry to build filed hospitals, buying personal protective equipment and scramble for ventilators reflected our lack of preparedness. Individual level preparedness is personal matter. Head of states, government officials increased awareness of risk. People focused on preparing for lock down, stocking up on food, medicine and supplies.

COVID is an excellent example of demonstration of death prevention behaviour. Because the condition gave a short term but intense risk of catching virus, there were very specific measures people could take to prevent the disease. Many countries, particularly Asia, wearing mask was not only acceptable in public places but was desirable. Again, element of denial, caused the Western countries to delay the advice. clearly, on live televised update, public health officials were admitting that wearing the mask would reduce the risk of asymptomatic patients transmitting the disease to the vulnerable. In the same update we were told the strategy is to reduce the transmission, mainly to the vulnerable group. In my humble opinion that translates to "wear the mask when you leave your home for any reason". But I am not a public health official. On individual level, social distancing and lockdown measures were part of prevention. People adhered to preventive measures largely, there were always some who thought otherwise. There always will be people who are attracted to risky behaviour, that is nihilistic pleasure and death instinct. I must pay tribute to all key workers, who knowing the risk well, went out to their jobs. That is some human quality above and beyond self-preservation. It is my personal belief that most people who voluntarily put themselves forward to help fellow men, lived a fulfilling life, the job they were doing was their fulfilment and meaning in life. That was their pathway in life.

PREMATURED UNTIMELY DEATH

People do die premature or untimely. We refer to a death as premature or untimely, when someone dies below expected average age of death or someone dies without an underlying illness which could cause death. Untimely death implies that person was not expected to die, or had a disease or incapacity which made death imminent. Perhaps numerically, the age of the dying person was below the mean or average age of death in the population. That is the problem with averages, if half of us live above average, other half have to die below average age.

What makes a premature death untimely, is total lack of death awareness, preparedness and acknowledgement of death as a possibility. At any given stage of the life cycle, it is easy to find reasons why you would not like to be death prepared. There could be younger dependents, a mortgage on the house, elderly parents, a business totally dependent on you or a loving partner you do not wish to see deprived of your relationship. But is event of the most unlikely, the life goes on and it has to go on. You can take some action, take some measures of death prevention and become aware of situations if untimely death occurs. You can facilitate the life of others to go on, without you. Not doing so, would be reflection of egocentric and selfish view about yourself.

SUMMARY

We all know we are going to die. But often we fail to remember it. It is the physical process of death which destroys us. The idea and thinking about it keeps us safe and makes us feel alive.

"I am not in denial, just I don't feel ready" – Author.

Pinnacle of Life

PLATONIC LOVE

I know you are there, somewhere in the abyss,

I am here, with open arms, waiting for the kiss.

In search of you everywhere, for a glimpse and smile,

I am prepared, aware, what bliss you can bring, from a mile.

My heart throbs, veins engorge, pulse raises by the thought,

Some time I lose sleep thinking I know you not.

Like marking of the wheels, on a wet muddy road,

our paths run parallel with pace of life, much in solitude.

I am sure one day you will change your course,

Will come close to me, to give me an embrace,

Take my breath, O dear death, be gentle and sweet,

When clock stops, I am all yours, when the parallel lines meet.

6 LONG LIFE AND IMMORTALITY

Every one wishes a long and healthy life. Long life is a practical desire. Not many thinks of being immortal, that is more religious and philosophical debate. Immortality is the indefinite continuation of a person's existence, even after death. It is virtually indistinguishable from afterlife, but philosophically speaking, they are not identical. Afterlife is the continuation of existence after death, regardless of whether or not that continuation is indefinite. Immortality implies a never-ending existence, regardless of whether or not the body dies. I recommend reading an amazing book, "immortality", The quest to live forever and how it drives civilisation, by Stephen Cave.

Advances in life style, preventive medicine, knowledge of causation of disease may have enabled people to live longer, but the fundamentals of biology of aging has not changed. There might be a multibillion cosmetic, surgical and food industry geared up to mask, slowdown and even rehabilitate age changes, but nothing, nothing stops the aging process. Every organ has its own aging pattern. Brain shrinks, arteries become stiffened, muscles waste, eye sight diminishes, teeth become prone to disease, glands dry up, and most importantly sensory and complex memory functions decline. To make up for each of the bodily changes, one adapts their daily activities. You can go for a walk rather than a run to make up for progressive loss of functional lung capacity. Have softer diet and derive more calories from simple carbohydrates rather than chewing prolonged period. Wear glasses, dentures, hearing aid, dye your hair and use mobility scooter. Perhaps a special enlarged display mobile with buttons is of some help. Stop multitasking and slow down the pace and variety of activities once we did without thinking about it. Taking regular medication may slow down the clogging of your arteries or bones getting thinner, but the pace and progression of aging process will catch up.

Aging is not just cumulative effect of wear and tear. Neither it is failure of our bodies repair system or genetic incapability to mend ourselves. Different organs age and fail with different mechanism. There is no singular cellular process to explain ageing. For all the claims we make about the advancement of science, the science has not improved the human life span, not even by a day. Genetically, physiologically and anatomically we are born and we die exactly same way as we did a centuries ago. What science has done is, it has prevented premature dying. It has stopped many people dying from disease until they achieve ripe old age. Science has not changed the aging process, not a bit. We still get older and fragile at the same rate as our ancestors did. What science has done, it has either provided an aid or substitute to mask the signs of ageing. Ageing process is unidirectional and cumulative.

However, as a result of prevention of premature death and help of masking ageing, people live longer, healthier and more productive than ever before. There are ever more exciting developments and interventions to help the aging population. More social care matters are now viewed as medical matters. There is also an unintended consequence of long life and highly mobile society. Longer you live, more isolated you are likely to be. Either you have lost friends and family or they live away from the place they were born. Reality is ever more than any time in history, people die in hospitals, hospices or care homes often not in presence of any relatives. Talking about one's end of life, their wishes and attending to their desires has never been more important.

DEATH EXPECTANCY

Normally described as life expectancy, is a quantitative measure of life span expectancy.

The term "life expectancy" refers to the number of years a person can expect to live. By definition, life expectancy is based on an estimate of the average age that members of a particular population group will be when they die. An important point to bear in mind when interpreting life expectancy estimates is that very few people will die at precisely the age indicated by life expectancy, even if mortality patterns stay constant. Maximum life span contrasts with mean life span (average life span, life expectancy), and longevity. Mean life span varies with susceptibility to disease, accident, suicide and homicide, whereas maximum life span is determined by "rate of aging". Longevity refers only to the characteristics of the especially long-lived members of a population, such as infirmities as they age or compression of morbidity, and not the specific life span of an individual. Since 1900 the global average life expectancy has more than doubled and is now above 70 years. The inequality of life expectancy is still very large across and within countries. In the early 19th century, life expectancy started to increase in the early industrialized countries while it stayed low in the rest of the world. This led to a very high inequality in how health was distributed across the world. Good health care was universal in the rich countries and persistently bad health in those countries that remained poor. Over the last decades this global inequality decreased.

Demographic research suggests that at the beginning of the 19th century no country in the world had a life expectancy longer than 40 years. A century ago, life expectancy in India and South

Korea was as low as 23 years. A century later, life expectancy in India has almost tripled and in South Korea it has almost quadrupled. The natural conclusion is that both advances of modern medicine and public health initiatives have helped us live longer than ever before, so much so that we may, in fact, be running out of innovations to extend life further. In September 2018, the Office for National Statistics confirmed that, in the UK at least, life expectancy has stopped increasing. Beyond the UK, these gains are slowing worldwide.

Life expectancy has been rising globally. However, this can be broken down further into 'healthy life expectancy' and 'years lived with disability'. It is true that there has been an increase for most countries in both aspects. Healthy life expectancy has increased across the world. It is also true that improved healthcare and treatments have also increased the number of years, on average, in which people live with a given disease burden or disability. In general, we tend to see that higher-income countries tend to spend more years with disability or disease burden than at lower incomes. In countries where the life expectancy is highest the expected years lived with disability or disease tend to be the longest too.

DEPENDENCE

Ageing of each organ and the functional adaptation eventually cumulates into change in way of life. For most people this, and not death, is the most fearful part of old age. We do not pay enough attention to the fact that at old age, day today help become necessity and life becomes dependent on this help. This brings about sense of loss of control, loss of independence and ability to make decisions on day to day basis. Unfortunately, in many cases, at this critical moment, people are forced to move away from their own homes into social and government funded care homes. This further enhances the anxiety and sense of loss of control. One can't avoid risk of becoming dependent at old age. You can delay it. People who are lonely become inactive and are at risk of becoming care dependent at early stage. In addition to decline in physical ability, cognitive decline, conditions like Alzheimer's disease can make people dependent. As a society, the care of the elderly is changing. It is also highly variable in different countries and cultures. Trend is for the families to become smaller and nuclear, and as a result older people tend not to live with or closer to their children. Also, modern society, mainly young people migrate readily following prospects of better jobs or opportunities, which again drives the families apart.

There always is hope, and there is. The science of communication over last decade has changed our way of life. We experienced this during lockdown period during the COVID pandemic. Online provides array of platforms to share every moment of life remotely at inexpensive way. Living remote somewhere in the world, if you have the right attitude, you can keep in touch with anyone in the world, anywhere relatively easily. I am not advocating that online contact substitute the human contact. However, hope is that the online contact tool promotes more human social interaction.

Care home and elderly care at home sector is well organised. However, the care setting is very expensive to run, often staffed by low paid but dedicated staff. Unless fundamental shift is social attitude towards funding occurs, the care home sector remains unaffordable for many in many countries. Longer life can also bring onset of many conditions affecting various parts of the body. This necessitates visit to the doctor more frequently, with more tests and interventions. In fact, this enhances the sense of dependency because elderly people rely on someone else to help them to travel to a medical facility.

IMMORTALITY

Humans throughout history have attempted to find that magic elixir which would enable to help them live longer or even forever.

China's first emperor ordered his subjects to search for the elixir of life in a quest for immortality. In fact, it is said that great wall of china was built to barricade death coming from unpredictable things from the north. First Emperor also sent a wise man, Xu Fu to find the elixir of immortality, who landed in japan and founded a new society proclaiming himself king. In 16th century France, nobles would drink gold in a bid to extend their lifespans. Gilgamesh, the Sumerian king at the heart of humanity's earliest epic poem, found a magic herb which would have given him an immortality, but a snake ate it. Hindu mythology describes "Amrut" an elixir came out of grand event of churning of the oceans. All the gods drank it and became immortals.

As Stephen Cave described in his book "Immortality", there are several paths mankind believed that the infinite life could be achieved. First the literal physical extension of life, just living longer. With advances in genetic therapy, preventive medicine and regenerative science, perhaps we can push the boundaries of human survival. We may be able to interfere in cellular age changes and enjoy youth for longer. The direction is established but no promise, even thought of an infinite life.

Second historical context is that of resurrection and being able to come back alive even after brief period of death. Biblical example of this is well known. Even in modern era, people have been brought back to life after period of death by cardio pulmonary resuscitation techniques. Perhaps freezing your DNA or genetic material, or even whole body (cryogenics), in a hope of resurrecting it in future belongs to this category.

Third is that of an essence of life, soul or atman, returning in another form or in another body thus the living element is recycled, and will remain infinite. Some religious teachings of reincarnation, rebirth, cyclical path of the soul allow humans to believe that the spirit is infinite. Some religions have described "Moksha" and "Nirvana" an end to the recycling of the spirit, and described integration of the soul with divine powers.

Fourth and perhaps the only effective way you can have longer life after death is the "Legacy" path. You die the last time when your name is spoken for the last time. Your deeds, actions and achievements remain in the mortal world long after you are gone. This also applies to your digital assets, social media accounts, collection of photographs and your favorite quotes and jokes as long as someone has remembered them. As we get older, we become more concerned for our legacy. Deep need to identify purpose of our life and making life worthwhile lead to the legacy path.

On the face of it, a desire for immortality most obviously seems to be a response to the fear of death. Most of us are afraid to die. If we were immortal, we could escape both that fear and its object. Hence, it seems, a desire for immortality is simply a desire not to die. In the face of this, what philosophers, poets and novelists remind us of is that there are fates worse than death. Immortality might itself turn out to be one of them. If so, we should not desire to be immortal.

In Jonathan Swift's satire Gulliver's Travels (1726), the protagonist meets the peculiar race of 'Struldbrugs', humans born with a strange mark on their foreheads, indicating that they will live forever. Initially thinking that these must be the happiest of all beings, Gulliver revises his view when he learns that Struldbrugs never stop ageing, leading them to sink into decrepitude and insanity, roaming the kingdom as disgusting brutes shunned by normal humans. Or consider Alfred, Lord Tennyson's poem Tithonus (1860), where an immortal narrator describes his physiological and psychological decay brought on by an endless life, and the horror and loneliness of being trapped in such a state.

THE WILL TO LIVE

The German philosopher **Arthur Schopenhauer** called the primary urge of live to extend living as "the will to live". Determination to survive and reproduce, and hence extend into the future, is one character all life forms have in common. Schopenhauer said the will is the subconscious force which drives every action of the conscious mind and blinds the intelligence. "By death, the individual achieves the peace of will-lessness, and finds salvation. Life laughs at the death of the individual, it will survive him in his offspring, or offspring of others. The satisfaction of the reproductive impulse is utterly and intrinsically reprehensible because it is the strongest affirmation of the lust for life". In our unconscious mind we do not believe that death can be caused by a natural cause. Hence death is always associated with a disease or a bad act, retribution, violence or punishment. The more we make progress in prevention, more will be the fear of dying.

Ever increasing life span is not good for the society. Older person working longer, denies a job and life opportunity for a younger one. Desperation to endlessly expand life is potentially expensive. Longer you live, more likely you are going to be incapacitated and dependent. Longer life, necessitates higher care and medical resources. And in countries where medical care is provided by the state, the burden of cost rises exponentially. Some kind of rationing has to apply, and often looser would be younger generation. Elderly care involves over use of diagnostic tests, widespread use of medication with unproven benefit and high cost. No wonder private care systems have hyped interest in promoting extreme elderly heath care. "disease awareness" is actively promoted, which intern promotes treatment awareness and cost. Increased spending on health care inevitably mean, for society and individual, we spend less on education, housing and transport. And again, likely affect is on younger generation.

Wisdom does not linearly increase with age forever! At some point in old age the brain starts to shrink, I don't mean you lose your wisdom but certainly you will start losing cognitive and intellectual capacity. Even if you manage to keep you brain well trained with all the sudoku puzzles you can find, body will start lagging behind. You have seen Gollum in Lord of the Ring. Eyes will need glasses, teeth replaced with implants, hips and knee with titanium as needed, and of course there are finest hearing aid and hair transplants as needed. I am not against medical devices or prosthetic procedures. I practice provision of them for living. But they should facilitate quality of life while living, not pretend to extend life itself.

LEGACY PATHWAY

Why should we think or care about our legacy? If you are

looking for meaning of life or purpose of your existence, legacy could be one of the answers. You would like to be remembered in the world by the living, when you are gone. We all know dinosaurs lived on the planet once and we know their legacy. We have some evidence, and digital recreations. We remember Shahjahan because history says he built Taj Mahal. There are grander schemes powerful men built on earth so that people could remember them. There are fortresses, paintings, scientific inventions, heroism and religions people started and we remember them, for a while at least. It may look very simple, but if you look at it philosophically, it is difficult to make any sense. There are two aspects for legacy or remembering. Who should remember you? And what should they remember.

Would you like to be remembered by your family members, people of your village or everyone in the world? For how long should they remember you? What should they remember? Your name or your picture, your stories or your memories? Take for example, Shahjahan built Taj mahal So that people would remember him and his wife Mumtaz. Yes, every time one visits Taj mahal they have been told that story, they perhaps think of Shajahan for a moment. But "Shahjahan" is just collection of alphabets, we know nothing more about him, even my name is collection of alphabets and so is yours. So, there is no realism in keeping your name alive for ever. Is it the physical body, preserved or a shrine you like as a memory? I travelled to Rome and wanted to see the place where the great Julius Ceaser was buried. And I did. Image of a lump heap of soil and some broken bricks and stone. Some dried flowers on top. Nothing would have given me enlightenment of mortality than sight of that grave. We all rest in same place, same destiny, no matter how heroic we act. Selfish motive should not be the reason for your legacy pathway.

Gratitude is the best way to design your legacy pathway. You owe everything to this planet, to your family and your society. Give something back. Look after the plane for the next generation, leave it as best state you can. That is the best legacy you can leave. Creating wealth, building towers and creating monuments at the expense of life of other people and the health of the plant should not be the goal. Sometimes donating blood, organs stem cells to help others live is seen as living through another person. It is a noble cause. Also remember every atom you are made up of will be recycled, and some day it will become part of some one's body, or will become part of body of something. That way your body is immortal.

DIGITAL LEGACY

We all leave behind digital traces when we are gone. Profiles, messages and images protected by passwords and encryption remain in web spaces after your life. The average person spends an essential part of their life on the internet and leaves a lot of sensitive information behind in the form of documents, files, images, videos, and much more. If someone dies unexpectedly, not only are they survived by those around them, but also by their online profiles and other content on the internet. For most online profiles, for example, it makes sense to deactivate them or turn them into memorial pages. However, bereavement also plays an important role in the death of a loved one who was very active on social media. Because an online profile continues to exist after the owner has died, it is still possible to interact with it. It makes sense to set an automatic reply for frequently used e-mail addresses so that the contact people know that the person they are trying to reach has died, and they can then be referred to another person if necessary.

The digital legacy becomes more complicated if the deceased person has been conducting business on the internet. Digital legacy is enormously important to influencers, content producers, and other people that make money online. Digital currency also needs to be managed. The gaming sector is also affected since content here (e.g. items in online games) can be worth real money. Only when you take a closer look at the subject, does it become clear how much data, accounts, profiles, and other digital possessions you actually own. If you don't manage your digital possessions effectively, you'll quickly overwhelm your heirs.

Depending on how carefully the digital legacy has been prepared, the heirs must first obtain an overview: Where was the deceased active on the internet? Which contracts did they finalise? Which data and possessions do they have stored online? Contracts should be terminated as soon as possible and profiles in social networks should be deactivated or deleted completely. Facebook, for example, also offers the option of converting the profile in question into a memorial page, but not every social network has this function. In most cases, you're advised to delete the profile. How easy this is depending on the network. With some providers, accounts can be deleted using a simple feature or a contact form, while others require proof of the user's death.

FINACIAL LEGACY

Also referred as inheritance, leaving behind your wealth to your family and dependents is a great endeavor. This will require careful planning and a lot of professional help is available. Knowing that the financial future of your family is safe after you are gone is one of the biggest considerations for many. This will reduce death anxiety significantly. It might not be easy but the satisfaction of knowing all your dedication has built a secure, promising and financially free future for your family is absolutely worth it.

What can you do to secure your family's financial future? First step, save while you are earning by living below your means. Aside from powering up the amount you can save, deep contentment can be found living a modest lifestyle. You don't get caught up trying to buy your way to happiness with material things. Pay off debts. Leaving behind debts in your estate can affect your family's finances hugely. Generally, loss of a person causes family additional burden of expenses such as funeral costs legal fees etc. you can really help your family by reducing the debt burden. Make sure you have adequate insurance and invest your savings wisely to create an income stream. Keep your legal documents and will up to date. Communicate with your family regularly about your finances. Estate planning is one of the best ways you can safeguard your property and leave behind something that all your coming generations can be proud of.

BEFORE YOU GO – SETTLE YOUR ACCOUNT

If you have a religious account, you may wish to settle it in your favor before you go. Many religions have prescribed way of doing this.

For Catholic believers, it is the last rite. The last rites are a religious process for cleansing sins before you leave this earth. Since Catholics believe in judgment after death, they want to leave this life as clean souls free from sin. The practice and prayers of the Last Rites protect the recipient on their journey to the afterlife. This is a type of Holy Communion given to someone who is dying. It also includes specific prayers and ceremonies. The Last Rights, or Viaticum, specifically refers to 3 sacraments. These are confession, the anointing of the sick, and final Holy Communion. Each of these is a way to cleanse a person's soul of sins in preparation for the afterlife.

In Islam, it is declaration of shahada, the confirmation of faith. When death approaches you, it is desirable on you to lie down on your back in such a way that the soles of your feet face the direction of Mecca. It is recommended to say by yourself or repeat after someone else the declaration of faith. This is a declaration in which you reconfirm your belief in Allah, Prophet Muhammad, the twelve Imams, the Quran, and the Day of Judgement. Followers of Hindu tradition believe in giving the dying person holy water from Ganges to wash away all the sins.

Everyone wants to set the account straight for their next world, but what about this world? I am sure we all owe something to this world, and what about settling your account here before your departure? Take time to think about your life time carbon foot print, resources exhausted in supplying you with food, shelter, clothing and comforts. What about that heap of plastic you are going to leave behind on this planet? We have a duty of care to this planet as much as you care about your next life. There are many ways you can settle this account. There is no magic prayer or holy water to fix that problem. Perhaps you can do a bit of DIY. Maybe you will remember this when you write your Will. Go to the fourth pillar of wisdom, write your own declaration of faithfulness to the planet. Plant a tree, clean up a beach, care for animals, stop using plastic, discourage buying of toxic chemicals. You know what is the best way you can settle your account.

SUMMARY

Immortality is fantasy. Even prolonged life may be not ideal. A balance is needed, and it is up to us as individuals to make a distinction between ideal life span and desired life span. Once you have decided how long is a desired life span for you, you can act of facilitating it. Of course, death takes no orders. Even though we have established there is no grim reaper, death can come to you any time.

DUALISM

Copernicus Galilei Newton and Bacon,

enlightened the mankind in darkness, with the beacon.

Hopes of new dawn of knowledge and sunshine,

Fresh look at life, release from biblical doctrine.

Out came Descartes, with mind and body dualism,

dashed the hopes of new dawn and mended the chasm,

Science gathered the 'matter', to split and grind,

religion strengthened it strangle hold on the 'mind'.

Death would have released the man and the mind,

all at once from the religious blind,

Cartesian dualism created two things from one,

Concept of soul, still lingers on, and is not gone.

7 CULTURE, CUSTOMS AND BELIEF.

As culturally diverse as the world is, there's so much to learn from each other about dying and grieving. Gaining a better understanding of the beliefs and practices of people around the world offers another way to connect and develop mutual respect for one another. I will not go into complete review of various cultural and religious belief around death and burial activity. I would like you to think about some issues with traditional practices like pollution, land usage, exploitation and see if alternate ways are feasible. Also, as a society we need to think if the celebration of death, should focus more on the life and contributions of the dead rather than addressing management of their soul.

There is a strong focus on religions because religion can be thought of as a cultural system of meaning that helps to solve problems of uncertainty, powerlessness, and scarcity that death creates. In placing death within a religious perspective, bereaved persons find meaning for an event that for many is inexplicable.

PHILIPPE ARIES

French historian Philippe Aries wrote several articles and a book titled "Western Attitudes Toward Death from the Middle Ages to the Present". The history of death was the subject of his work in his last decade of scholarly life.

In his first chapter, he discusses the first period, "Tamed Death", using a number of ancient texts and medieval romances. He argues that prior to the seventeenth century, people were acutely aware of their own imminent death, prepared for it, and accepted it. Rituals were often religious such as positioning the body to be facing Jerusalem. The dying man readied his body and soul for death and waited. There were four general characteristics: first, the dying person would usually be lying in bed, or at least in a recumbent position. In the Christian tradition the dying person would lie on his or her back, facing the heavens. Second, the dying person in this period always presided over his death and understood its accompanying religious rituals and protocol. The priest was not brought until he was called for, and loved ones did not say goodbye until the dying person consented. Third, death was a public ceremony and parents, spouses, family, neighbors and even children were present at the bedside. Death was seen as normal and it was customary for loved ones to witness the occasion. Finally, while accepted and witnessed, it lacked "theatrics" and a "great show of emotions". Ariès, explains his choice of "Tamed Death" as a title is meant to contrast with the "wild" death of the twentieth century, in which people fear and avoid death.

Subtle changes in western people's attitudes toward death occurred around the eleventh and twelfth centuries. Ariès titled this mentality shift: "One's Own Death". The defining feature of this era was a new personalization of death, in which the individual rather than the act of death itself came to the forefront. By the twelfth century Ariès observes that Last Judgment had taken on new meaning. It came to signify judgment passed on one's soul after the moment of death. In the new Christian tradition, people believed that after death their good and bad deeds would be weighed against each other, and based on those deeds they would be either dammed or admitted immediately into heaven. This made death more personal and individual. Ariès notes that the actual moment of death began to gain greater significance, as Christians believed that a person's deathbed behaviour and personal reflection on their own deeds, at the moment of death, could influence heavenly judgment. As in the previous era friends and family were often present, but their presence became more closely tied to witnessing the moment before judgment rather than simply witnessing death. In this era, depictions of corpses and skeletons became more prevalent, and individual tombs with inscriptions grew in popularity. Although religious artwork had featured macabre themes in the past, by the seventeenth century there was an influx of artwork that featured decaying cadavers and the physical body after death.

By the early eighteenth century, Ariès observed an abrupt change in the western person's attitude toward death. Death was dramatized, exalted, feared, and in some cases worshipped. People did not look at death as a familiar occasion that was part of life, as they had in the past. Although people continued to participate socially and ritualistically in death, and crowds still flocked to the bedside of a dying person, their purpose had changed. Instead of witnessing death, they mourned it. Ariès argues that it became unregulated. It was less of a ritualized social obligation, and more of a spontaneous and often excessive display of emotions. Ariès maintains that survivors no longer accepted the death of friends and loved ones. He states that people of this period lamented that death was such a complete rupture from life and were consoled by preserving the memory of the deceased. Memorializing the dead became an important feature of the period of "thy death".

The final period Ariès demarcates in the evolution of western attitudes toward death is the era of "forbidden death". Beginning in the very late nineteenth and early twentieth centuries, Ariès argues that a "brutal revolution" occurred in western attitudes toward death, in which death became both shameful and forbidden. Growing out of the sentimental era of "thy death" in which survivors mourned the death of loved ones openly, spontaneously, and with heightened displays of emotion, it soon became common practice to shield the people actually dying from the reality of their condition. The mourner, so moved by the gravity of death, wished to spare their dying loved one any emotional turmoil. Thus, in the era of "forbidden death" the dying man no longer presided over his own death. Soon the extreme emotions that survivors expressed in the previous period were replaced with an equally extreme avoidance of death and suppression of emotion that became dominant in twentieth century. Ariès names two societal trends that he believes were very influential on shifting attitudes toward death: the advent of the hospital as a place of dying, and a growing sentiment that life should be, above all, happy.

QUE SERA SERA - ATTITUDES TOWARDS DEATH

"Que sera sera, whatever will be, will be" is probably best summary of our modern attitude towards death. The attitude towards death is the function of the individual psychological development. This is dependent on the level of social development and scientific knowledge. What makes a difference in the inevitability of death is usually the belief and attitude towards it. Among different societies of the world, how, when, where and what can cause death had become a source of concern to individuals, groups and even specialists such as Psychologists, Sociologists, Social workers etc., world over. There is evidence that divergence in culture, life experience and civilization can significantly affect the way individuals and groups can perceive death and dying. In any case we are unlikely to develop independent thinking towards death, either we pretend ignorance and sing que sera sera or put responsibilities on someone else saying "Will of God or Insha Allah".

In African traditional societies, death is attached with sacredness. Often death is believed to have been caused by supernatural powers. It is harder for people to see death as natural phenomenon. In the understanding of majority of traditional African people, it is assumed that death before certain age in life is unnatural and therefore is connected to invisible powers. This attitude to death has done more harm than good to the families and households even communities where such attitude is dominant. In most societies in Africa especially in Nigeria rural communities, there is a lot of bitterness which is overtly or covertly shown after burial. In most cases, some individuals or even families have to avoid the burial scene reasons ranging from the fear of being accused to some people avoiding being bewitched at the arena. Out of fear, some people decide to leave the community during the burial to avoid trouble. In most cases, such deliberate avoidance is interpreted as tacit signs of guilt, and the houses and other personal belongings of such people are often destroyed. Belief and attitude towards death and dying is a subject to experience from the environment and culture in which one lives. By implication, what people show as attitude towards death and dying is typically the reflection of his cultural background including religious belief.

Referencing anthropologist Geoffrey Gorer, Ariès states that death has replaced sex as western society's greatest taboo. Children are less likely to be shielded from the notion of sex in the modern era, but they are not taught about death.

To know what dying means to you, you must know what living means to you. If your living identity is some or all of things like work, office, family, relationship, hopes, fears, pleasure, intellect and knowledge, then that is your identity. Death is the end to all that identity. Life may be hard and living may be a struggle. To stay alive, earn a livelihood, try to be moral and try to be good to others may appear hard, but we cling to that struggle, because we know the living. In death there may be security, permanence, indestructability and peace, but we do not want to think about it because it is the unknown.

CUSTOMS AND EXPLOITATION

"Nisha was devastated at the events of her father's death she was at home anticipating this was going to happen. Her family had done everything they felt appropriate to keep her dad comfortable through his last days. He had discussed with them about his wishes, what he would be remembered for and how he was proud and happy to be the man he was. According to the Hindu custom, her father's body was cremated.

Nisha's father was not a religious man, she wasn't even sure he really believed in god. But he was a kind, generous and helpful person and participated in every social and community events. When these events were in local temple. he would visit them and take part in prayers as a communal event. Other than this, there was no involvement of religion in Nisha's upbringing.

A family elder turned up at her house day after the funeral, with a priest. He introduced the priest as the best in the area for rituals performed after cremations, the "Uttar kriya". The priest spoke in length how he can help her dad's soul to achieve ultimate release from rebirth cycles, and find him a place in heaven. Her family were vulnerable, and in no position to reject this offer of help. Nor they wished to upset the family elders who were trying to help. The priest settled down with his book, noted the precise moment of death, direction of the body at the time of death and other details he thought were important. He proclaimed that the death had happened at a difficult junction of stars, but he can fix that with a special offering. He suggested the family should donate some land, gold and a cow to the local temple. The ceremony would take place on the twelfth day of the death, when the should would leave this world and transcend to a higher level. Nisha's mum agreed to this arrangement though it would cost lot of her savings.

List of auxiliary items needed for the ceremony kept growing, so did the cost. A feast for all the family and friends was followed by generous gifts to all priests attended the ceremony. Visit to the town of Varanasi, to scatter the ashes in river Ganga, a thirty days daily prayer and lamp decoration in the temple did not come at low cost. Further there were incidental expenses, ex on the twelfth day ceremony, a crow did not appear quick enough to eat the offering. So, the priest asked the family to make a special offering of forgiveness. Eventually a crow appeared, and bit into a ball of rice kept on a banana leaf outside the house. Priest explained that this was a sign that her father's soul has now left for a good place and all his efforts have been successful. Even though, it left her in debt, Nisha's mum was satisfied that everything was done appropriately to help her husband. Nisha was left dismayed by the power of established religious and cultural system, which would readily exploit people's feeling to make profit. The priest would move on to help another soul, departed in some other part of the town. The culture of donating cows, clothes, gold and pieces of land continues."

BURIAL RITUALS AND FUNERAL

The established practice of saying final goodbye to a person is often formal, religious or cultural ceremony. Many of such events focus on the death and reinforcing beliefs of life cycles and reincarnations rather than celebrating the life of the person. Hymns and chants describe the role of supernatural powers to release the dead persons soul and give it a peaceful afterlife. Often people praise and bribe these powers, trying to influence them to get the best, most revered position to the dead.

Wouldn't it be more relevant, if the nurse who cared for you in your last days, the work colleague who has been with you in difficult times, and your childhood friends played a major role in your funeral service. Not all services of death need to somber or sad with sense of loss. The life of the person who lived a meaningful life, had a peaceful end, contributed to everyone else around them, should be celebrated and not mourned.

Regardless of variations in conceptions and attitudes toward death, ceremonies provide survivors a sense of closure after a loss. These rites and ceremonies send the message that the death is real and allow friends and loved ones to express their love and duty to those who die. Under circumstances in which a person has been lost and presumed dead or when family members were unable to attend a funeral, there can continue to be a lack of closure that makes it difficult to grieve and to learn to live with loss. And although many people are still in shock when they attend funerals, the ceremony still provides a marker of the beginning of a new period of one's life as a survivor.

White is the colour of mourning in China, not black, as in the west, and as such, is regarded as unlucky; this is why giving white flowers to a Chinese person is inappropriate. Funeral rituals vary according to the age and status of the deceased but the official mourning period for a Buddhist may go on for 100 days. These rituals are elaborate and may even include hiring professional wailers, in the belief that the young in China no longer know how to show emotion appropriately. Japan is the opposite. Death is seen as liberation and acceptance is more important than expressing oneself. People bring condolence money to wakes in white envelopes tied with black and white ribbon.

Muslims bury their dead, rather than cremate them, in the belief that there will be a physical resurrection on the Day of Judgment. The dead are buried facing Mecca and graves raised above the ground, or marked by stones, so nobody walks on them. Because the death of a Muslim is regarded as a loss to the Muslim community overall, it is not uncommon for people who did not even know the deceased to attend funerals. A mourning period of up to 40 days follows a burial.

In the Hindu faith, it is preferable to die at home, surrounded by family. The soul is believed to go on, according to one's karma. Bodies are cremated quickly, usually within 24 hours, in order to liberate the soul quickly. Mourners wear white, not black, and people do not bring food to the wake, but to a ceremony 13 days after the cremation, at which the soul is liberated and the mourning period considered over. Ashes are scattered over water, the most desirable place being the holy Ganges and a lot of Hindu families living outside India will make the pilgrimage to do this. Tibetan sky burials leave the deceased's body on a platform for vultures to eat. After the funeral, the deceased's soul arrives in Paradise.

MEMORIALS

Building of personal memorials or monuments is a symbolic gesture towards immortality. Urge to leave behind monuments is more generally symbolic of desire to leave behind a mark to be remembered. Gathering material riches to pass down is sign of this. Parents entering into guiding their children is also a form of monumentalism.

In this early medieval period people were not concerned with what would happen to their bodies after death. For superstitious reasons they did not want the dead to be buried in cities or near the houses of the living, but if the body was buried in a churchyard and remained under the church's protection, little else mattered.

Pinnacle of Life

In Korea, where cremation is becoming commonplace nowadays, there is a trend to have the ashes of a loved one refined and turned into colourful beads. While these are not worn, if you visit a Korean home and see these beads on display, they're likely to be the ashes of a loved one of the home owner.

Gone but not forgotten, you'll find information about memorials erected to the dead all around the world, including war memorials in the United States and controversial memorials in Ireland. The Spanish monuments in California draw large crowds annually. Some cultures set aside days annually to honour the dead, such as Memorial Day in the United States.

EXPRESSION OF GRIEF

Many cultures express grief in rather creative ways, including through poetry or music. For some, following specific traditions when it comes to burial and grieving brings comfort to those left behind, such as the death rituals of the Jewish people or the Buddhist people. Specific garments can signify a: In some cultures, showing grief, including wailing, is expected of mourners because the more torment displayed and the more people crying, the more the person was loved. In other cultures, restraint is expected. Rules in Egypt and Bali, both Islamic countries, are opposite; in Bali women may be strongly discouraged from crying, while in Egypt women are considered abnormal if they don't nearly incapacitate themselves with demonstrative weeping. In Japan, it is extremely important not to show one's grief for a number of reasons. Death should be seen as a time of liberation and not sorrow, and one should bear up under misfortune with strength and acceptance. One never does anything to make someone else uncomfortable. In Latino cultures, it may be appropriate for women to wail, but men are not expected to show overt emotion due to "machismo." In China, hiring professional wailers may be customary in funerals, which may sound odd, but this was also a common practice in Victorian England as an expression of grief, such as the mourning bonnets worn by women in the Civil War era.

CELEBRATION OF THE DEAD

Mode of music represents mood of mind in public gatherings. Jazz bands accompanying funeral marches in New Orleans do lift the spirit of the mourners and give celebratory tone to the march. Accompanied by dancing, the atmosphere is conducive to keep good memories of the diseased person.

Ghana is another example of this belief in an afterlife, with a relatively new tradition of elaborate coffins, which will illustrate the interests, profession or status of the departed but also see them off into the next life in style. A coffin may take the form of an aeroplane, or a Porsche, or a Coca Cola bottle, an animal or even, in dubious taste, a giant cigarette packet. Coffin makers are highly sought after and are regarded as important artists. Funerals are enormous affairs, often costing more than weddings, and advertised on huge billboards so that nobody in the community misses out.

The premise of ancestor worship is based on understanding that the course of life is cyclical not linear. Those who are dead may not be seen physically, but are alive in a different world and/or can reincarnate in new births. Ancestor worship in various forms can be found in many parts of the world and is very strong in parts of Africa and Asia. Many Native Americans and Buddhists alike believe that the living co-exist with the dead. A central theme in all ancestor worship is that the lives of the dead may have supernatural powers over those in the living world –

the ability to bless, curse, give or take life. In some cultures, worship of the dead is important, and includes making offerings of food, money, clothing, and blessings. In China there is the annual observance of "sweeping the graves" and as its name denotes, it is a time for people to tend the graves of the departed ones. In Mexico, there is The Day of the Dead (Dia de los Muertos), a holiday that focuses on gatherings of family and friends to pray for and remember those who have died. The Day of the Dead is also celebrated by many Latin Americans living in the U.S. and Canada. The intent of the celebration is to encourage visits by the souls of the departed so that those souls will hear the prayers and the comments of the living directed at them. It makes sense that in cultures where ancestor worship is common, the acceptance of organ donation and cremation may be low.

Countries like Costa Rica, Panama, and Guatemala show the importance of family in life and death. Immediate and extended family members provide comfort and aid in grief. Latinos don't shy away from discussions of death. First, the family holds a vela or celebration for the deceased in countries like Nicaragua and Costa Rica. Guests drink alcohol and eat pastries as they stay up all night, sharing memories of their loved ones.

The majority of people living in the Middle East believe in the religion of Islam. Muslim funerals are simple and focus on the deceased's actions in the earthly realm. Families show emotion openly, often screaming, crying, or slapping their faces. Islamic funerals are the opposite of the Latin celebrations or African worship. Muslims are uniquely united in death. Family, friends, and neighbors gather together to bring food to the deceased's family and share in prayer. Only God knows the timing of each Muslim's death, and each Muslim has a set time they will pass into the afterlife. To reach the afterlife, Muslims have to follow Islamic laws based on the holy Quran. Finally, death isn't an easy process either; it's bitter and painful for Muslims, especially the soul separating from the body. People all over the Middle East unite over religious customs. It's an integral part of Middle Eastern culture.

UNFAMILIAR CULTURAL BELIEFS

For health care professionals, providing culturally sensitive bereavement/end of life care is understandably an issue of discomfort. Language and cultural barriers obviously compound the challenges of being professionally appropriate and compassionate. Patients and families may be in need of compassion, advice, and guidance from doctors and nurses, but often the realities of a given situation include a press for time and both physical and emotional exhaustion among providers and families. It happens – sometimes we simply fail, in the moment, to express sufficient sensitivity and warmth when critical decisions must be made. The clinical facts are immediate and demand logical linear thinking which is natural for those trained in the Western medical tradition. For many cultures, such a direct approach may seem harsh, and decisions about something like organ donation might be experienced as inhumane immediately upon death. The questions suggested in this article can be used to ease some of the communication challenges and facilitate more openness between health care professionals and families around death and dying. Of course, they should be tailored to the context of a given situation.

Death is universal and every culture has its own ways of dealing with it. From how a person is laid to rest to how he is memorialized, every culture and religion has a unique way of burying, grieving and memorializing their deceased ones. Explore cultural views on death and dying, as well as particular customs that make each one unique.

HUMOUR AND DEATH

Death is no fun. It is a very sensitive and delicate subject and a very emotionally charged time for everyone involved. So, humour and death do not mix well. However psychologically we derive some relief in witnessing death when it happens to someone else. It is a way to offset your own anxiety about death. Also, humans have attraction to Thanatos or even homicidal tendencies in humour often termed as black humor. Some jokes release such subconscious thoughts. A lady says to her friend "My husband is an Angel". Friend replied "You lucky devil, mine is still alive".

The joke of the clown in a retirement home has the same reflection. When asked, "Are all of you here?" the elderly reply "yes" and clown adds "but not for long". Humour helps people to cope. It empowers them to be defiant and provide perspective and balance. George Bernard Shaw said "Life does not cease to be funny when people die, any more than it ceases to be serious when people laugh!"

Studies have long shown that people who laugh have a more positive outlook on life. But what about people facing death or their relatives? Can we manage pain physically and the pain feeling of losing someone better with layer of humour? Humour can certainly help to share the positivity, a well lived life and all the joy rather than focus on the impending loss. Also, good humour in the days leading to death can be great memories and you can go back to them again as a way of remembering the person. Humour is not a solution to grief nor it is cure for the death. But it has the potential to open the door of emotions, which we can share. Humour is also a way of mocking death and I certainly hope my end will be surrounded by plenty of humour.

SUMMARY

What Are Your Final Wishes?

Now that we've travelled around the world exploring death perspectives, you can begin thinking of your own funeral wishes. Is your death view religious or secular? Think about how you would like to be remembered—a gravestone isn't the only option (you can plant a tree instead!) From burial to legal planning—it can be overwhelming to think of your death. Cake can help. Your end-of-life planning profile stores your wishes so you can share them with friends and family and fully live in the present.

CARE HOME

This is my home, filled with love and care,

Porridge, sponge bath and they shampoo my hair,

I have rules to follow, when I can be seen,

Four walls tell me, I should have structure to my routine.

It is my body that needs caring, my mind is set free,

My sight isn't clear, there is always sun for me to see.

Am a bit hard of hearing, but listen Robin chirping, not shy,

Oh, a butterfly I can't chase, I forget, I could never fly.

I think world is my home, there will be no walls,

when my thoughts are set free, there will be no falls.

Grateful I lived in this body all my life,

gracefully let me make my way back,

Like dvaita and dualism dictate for end of any creature,

return my mind to mystery and body to the nature.

8 CARE AND CURE

At some stage in progression of human life, there will come a point where one has to make a decision to continue or limit the medicalisation of life. Illness or deterioration has cumulative effect, so is ageing. Person may decide not to have certain treatment or procedure, even though there is reasonable amount of successful outcome, for various reasons. Some people worry that they may not be able to make or convey their decision in the end, and hence wish to execute a decision in advance. Others may not be willing to go through the suffering and ill health.

Social factors also play a role in end of life decision making process. In traditional culture, and some eastern societies, it is still expected norm that older people take significant role in running of the society. As village elderly, teachers of tradition and guardians of cultural values, older people feel valued, and listened to. Many times, they take role of arbitration, judiciary, religious guide, confidants and enforcers of belief and customs. That role has been discarded in individualist, nuclear family based cultures. Often old people are lonely, disempowered actively and they see life and lifestyle changing every day without any say in it. This may lead to people losing the will of life and a desire to carry on. Social recognition of this is needed. I am focusing on a small element of this social phenomenon related to end of life. Providing a reassurance to the growing old that they will be cared for at the end of life is an essential duty. There are some ways we can empower the elderly in relation to end of life.

ADVANCED CARE DIRECTIVE

An advance care directive is a person's oral or written instructions about his or her future medical care, if he or she becomes unable to communicate. It may be in written or oral form. It may also contain the names of persons to make decisions on a person's behalf, on what kind of treatment would be desirable, in situations that the person concerned may be incapable of making such decisions personally. This affords individuals the opportunity to exercise their rights regarding their medical care in advance. It is popular in most western countries. However, the advanced care directive need not be documented, legal text or formal instruction. With death awareness and an ability to talk about one's own death, wishes could be expressed in any form.

In some countries, an advance directive is a legal document. It tells your doctor and family what kind of medical care you want to have if you can't tell them yourself. This could happen if you are in are in a coma, are seriously injured, are terminally ill or develop severe dementia. If you are admitted to the hospital, the hospital staff will probably talk to you about advance directives.

A good advance directive describes the kind of treatment you would want, depending on how sick you are. It could describe what kind of care you want if you have an illness that you are unlikely to recover from. It could also describe the care you want if you are permanently unconscious. Advance directives usually tell your doctor that you don't want certain kinds of treatment. They can also say that you want a certain treatment no matter how ill you are. A living will is one type of advance directive.

POWER OF PROXY ON HEALTH

As we approach end stage of life, both physical and psychological strain may not allow us to make decisions. Many people rely of family members to make best care decisions on their behalf. Recognise, that it is very hard for family to make rational decision in the emotionally demanding time. Also, people with a group like families may have varying opinion and this may cause difficulty in arriving at a decision, can cause rift withing the group. It is therefore advisable to appoint single person with authority to make decision on your behalf. This person could be a family member, medical practitioner, a legal attorney or a hospital appointed champions.

A durable power of attorney (DPA) for health care is another kind of advance directive. A DPA states whom you have chosen to make health care decisions for you. It becomes active any time you are unconscious or unable to make medical decisions (and may be called Medical Power of Attorney, or MPOA). A DPA is generally more useful than a living will. But a DPA may not be a good choice if you don't have another person you trust to make these decisions for you.

Physician orders for life-sustaining treatment (POLST) is for people who have been diagnosed with a serious illness. It is filled out by your doctor. It doesn't replace your other advance directives. Instead it stays with you to ensure you get the medical treatment you want.

Do not resuscitate order (DNR) order can also be part of an advance directive. Hospital staff try to help any patient whose heart has stopped or who has stopped breathing. They do this with cardiopulmonary resuscitation (CPR). A DNR is a request not to have CPR if your heart stops or if you stop breathing.

You can use an advance directive form or tell your doctor that you don't want to be resuscitated. Your doctor will put the DNR order in your medical chart. Doctors and hospitals in all states accept DNR orders. They do not have to be part of a living will or another advance directive.

Other possible end-of-life issues that may be covered in an advance directive include, Ventilation if, and for how long, you want a machine to take over your breathing, Tube feeding , if, and for how long, you want to be fed through a tube in your stomach or through an IV. And palliative care (comfort care) keeps you comfortable and manages pain. This could include receiving pain medicine or dying at home.

Even if you are in good health, you might want to consider writing an advance directive. An accident or serious illness can happen suddenly. If you already have a signed advance directive, your wishes are more likely to be followed. In the African culture, the elderly or aged may give verbal instructions to their children concerning their care at the end of their lives. Such instructions may include avoiding prolonged hospital stay, allowing them to die on their own beds and in their children's arms at home, how to conduct the burial ceremony, where they are to be buried. Cultural and spiritual beliefs tend to make individuals, especially the middle-aged ones, avoid making end-of-life decisions while still alive and young.

EUTHANASIA

Euthanasia is considered to be *voluntary* when it takes place in accordance with the wishes of a competent individual, whether these wishes have been made known personally or by a valid advance directive—that is, a written statement of the person's future desires in the event that he or she should be unable to communicate his or her intentions in the future. A person is considered to be competent if he or she is deemed capable of understanding the nature and consequences of the decisions to be made and capable of communicating this decision. An example of voluntary euthanasia is when a physician gives a lethal injection to a patient who is competent and suffering, at that patient's request.

Arguments in favour of euthanasia are generally based upon beliefs concerning individual liberty, what constitutes a "good" or "appropriate" death, and certain life situations that are considered unacceptable. These arguments are generally based upon moral or religious values as well as certain beliefs concerning the value and quality of human life. They also often suppose that people are capable of making rational decisions, even when they are suffering and terminally ill.

The arguments against euthanasia include religious and ethical beliefs about the sanctity of life as well as a number of arguments allowing for euthanasia that will inevitably lead to a situation where some individuals will risk having their deaths hastened against their will.

SUICIDE – SELF EUTHANASIA

Common sense would say that self-killing must be the ultimately disadvantageous act, a sure path to genetic oblivion. When someone kills them self in order to remove their bodily person from the world, it would seem quite plausible that they believe the knock-on effects will improve things for others. This is altruistic suicide.

The common goal of suicide is cessation of consciousness. The idea of cessation that you can be free of all your problems, get out of this mess, cancel your debts, release yourself from this anguish, stop this disease is the turning point in the suicide. Given their insight that killing themselves will put an end to their suffering, suicide can seem to provide a perfectly rational solution: a reliable method of *self-euthanasia*. Nothing hurts less than being dead.

Abrahamic religions, in particular, make a point of threatening that the afterlife for sinners, and suicides especially, will be an unpleasant one. Idea of a horrible afterlife was never invented specifically to deter suicide. But if, as is surely the case, it has consistently worked to this effect, this is presumably a reason why it has taken such a hold.

People kill themselves 'when they want to go', sometimes after careful reflection, sometimes on the spur of the moment, sometimes for profound reasons and sometimes for shallow ones. Hamlet asks *'who would bear the whips and scorns of time, the oppressor's wrong, the proud man's contumely, the pangs of despised love, the law's delay, the insolence of office, and the spurns that patient merit of the unworthy takes, when he himself could his quietus make with a bare bodkin?'* The answer is, evidently, by no means everyone.

VOLUNTARY STOPPING OF EATING AND DRINKING (VSED)

To voluntarily stop eating and drinking means to refuse all food and liquids, including those taken through a feeding tube, with the understanding that doing so will hasten death. This is an option for people with terminal or life-limiting diseases who feel that with VSED their dying will not be prolonged. One of the advantages of this decision is that you may change your mind at any time and resume eating and drinking. Talk with friends and family members who might care for you during this process early about your wishes and why you may want to take this course. Their support is crucial. Complete an Advance Directive stating in writing that voluntarily stopping eating and drinking is your wish. Have your physician sign orders to withhold life-sustaining therapies and all resuscitation efforts.

The cessation of eating and drinking is a normal part of the dying process, and is usually very peaceful, without a sense of hunger or thirst. People may choose to stop eating and drinking as a way to have some control over their death. This decision can generate mixed emotions, but the bottom line is that when death occurs after a person stops eating and drinking it does not occur because of starvation or dehydration. It occurs because of the underlying medical condition responsible for the dying process. In this setting, not eating may hasten death somewhat, but usually involves very little suffering. Most often, the voluntary stopping of eating and drinking results in a peaceful death which honours the person's last wishes.

SAYING GOOD BYE

Saying good-bye is not easy. Yet, it is important for the dying person and his/her loved ones to do so. Take advantage of opportunities when the person is awake and communicative to facilitate the "**saying good-bye**" process.

If the dying person is not lucid, or in a coma, remember that hearing is the last sense to leave. Assume everything you say can be heard and understood, even if the person is not responsive. Never speak about the dying person as if he was not in the room. Some people feel comfortable lying in bed next to their loved one as they say their parting words. Others may want to simply hold hands. If music, chanting, or prayer is used to assist the dying, let it be comforting and familiar, making way for gentle passage. The dying person's body language will let you know if these sounds are welcome and soothing.

Even with all the preparation and knowledge that death is coming, the moment of death is not easy to see. Some education about expected events like change in breathing sound, gasping and other events, may reduce the uncomfortable situation for the family present at the time. It is like being aware of what to expect at child birth. Even those people who are closest to the dying person may choose to be absent. The decision to be present at the moment of death depends on many things.

Inability to say goodbye was one of the major issues with COVID pandemic associated deaths. In United Kingdom, midway through the pandemic, health secretary made provisions to supply infection control provisions to relatives so that they can say goodbye in controlled isolated environment. In particular this problem was affecting care home sector when dying long term residents could not be seen by relatives because strict preventive guidelines on visits. In addition, once patients were ill at the level requiring intensive care treatment, the system was so inundated that relatives could not keep contact with the patient. Many only saw them if they made through it. I do not know if it is true, when communicable diseases hit villages in India, a century ago, I was told that affected patients were carried to temple buildings outside the village and left there with some basic needs. This was done to prevent spread of the disease to rest of the village. Patients either died, or walked back to the village if they got better. With pandemic, we succeeded in sedation, oxygen and ventilation, but often failed the relatives to alleviate their anxiety.

WHAT DOCTORS DO NOT KNOW

Doctors are very good about knowing the disease. Many know the best way to treat the disease. But they know very little about you. It is impossible for a doctor to know what is best for you. In fact, only you know what is best for you. Concept of family doctor, who knew more about you due to long term practice and continuity of care, is slowly disappearing form medical world. Due to regulations and overseeing needs, it is likely that you will see multiple medical professionals. Also, extreme specialisation in medical field, means one specialist only deals with one aspect of your ailment.

Many consultations I do only last 15 minute. At best I am more or less restricted to doing an examination and discuss one result or advice some test. The focus is always on cure rather than care.

There is also an ethical issue of over medicalisation. This can happen from a combination of over diagnosis and over treatment. Overdiagnosis is a correct diagnosis, but the treatment is unlikely to benefit the person. This can be driven by increased sensitivity of the tests, finding things which we were not looking for and also expanded definition of the disease and lowering thresholds. Sometimes, fear of missing a diagnosis leads to creation of a diagnosis. There is also public and political enthusiasm for a specific diagnostic process like screening, which encourages policy makers to over drive the process. Obviously, there is financial and commercial interest affecting some medicalisation. There should be a pill for every ill and not an ill for every pill.

BREAKING (BAD) NEWS

Bad news may be defined as "any information which adversely

and seriously affects an individual's view of his or her future". The task of breaking bad news can be improved by understanding the process involved and approaching it as a stepwise procedure, applying well-established principles of communication.

A lady had left her cat and dog in an animal care center while on holiday. She called the center to enquire if they were all right. The manager took the call said "sorry madam your cat is dead". She was very upset, not because of the death of her cat but because of the bluntness in which the news was delivered. She knew her cat was terminally ill. She complained "you could have been more subtle, you could have said, it was playing on the roof garden, and had a minor fall, you could have delayed may be for a day to say you gave it the best treatment and care, and may be a day later you should have broken the news gently to say in spite of your best care, the cat died, and how sorry you were". The manager agreed. "She carried on "by the way how is my dog". The manager hesitated, "he, he is playing on the roof garden, madam, please call tomorrow and I will update".

Medical professionals and relatives often have to update ill person or relatives about new changes in the medical situation. The message has to be specific but delivered in a way, it is clearly understood. However often the question is around information that is impossible to give.

It was my job to deliver "bad news" to an elderly gentleman. As a trainee, I followed every single step of my protocol to ensure, I had delivered the news correctly. "I wish I could tell you different, but the MR image confirms size of the tumour next to your major blood vessel. It is not treatable" "So I am going to die?" I replied "yes", with correct body posture, tone, and closer distance to the gentleman as per protocol. He laughed "I knew that", I asked how, "you only came with shoulder pain?" he replied "doctor, I also know you are going to die" It was my turn to feel dizzy. "have you ever met a man who is not going to die?" he asked. We both laughed for a brief moment. "I don't suppose you know when I am going to die" he asked. "roughly may be few months, may be even longer, or it could even be sooner" I realised I was not doing well. Gentleman wished me all the best with my training before he left the room.

Updating health issues, in particular, results which indicate further progress of disease and life limitation is stressful. However, creating false hope of hiding information is also not ethical and often not helpful. Awareness and acceptance are the key.

CARING FOR PERSON FACING DEATH.

The more people engage and understand death and know where it's heading, the better prepared the person is to be able to let go to the process, and the better prepared the family is to reconcile with it, for a more peaceful death. Of course, not everyone ends up in palliative care or even in a hospital. For some people, death can be shockingly sudden, as in an accident or from a cardiac arrest or massive stroke. Death can follow a brief decline, as with some cancers; or a prolonged one, as with frailty; or it can come after a series of serious episodes, such as heart failure. And different illnesses, such as dementia and cancer, can also cause particular symptoms prior to death.

An old man visited his wife at a care home every day. She was suffering from advanced dementia and did not recognise him, and at times was abusive. The manager of the nursing home was talking to the old man one day, asked him, why he would visit her every day, while she does not remember or recognise him anymore. The man replied "but I still remember who she is"

Of course, dying people need appropriate physical pain control.

But they also have needs to feel heard, cared-for, connected and emotionally safe. Dying people want to be understood and accepted like anyone else. The most important thing you can give to a dying person is to listen. When communicating with a dying person, be respectful. We do not know what patient's belief is about death and after death experience, and it is important not to force our viewpoint onto the person. Often in difficult situations we tend to deny what's happening, or make a joke of it. While such reactions are very normal, dying is a profound process that just needs us to be there, and perhaps hold a hand. It is perhaps more important to engage in body language and expression than what you actually say. You may feel fearful of seeing your relative become helpless and vulnerable. Try to stay calm. Don't feel you have to talk all the time. Just being there quietly at the bedside is important, and can often be surprisingly peaceful. Dying people often feel compelled to confront and resolve unfinished issues from their past, particularly with family members. They may want to write a letter or send an email, or meet with the person in question. They may also have a desire to visit childhood haunts or go through old family photographs. These experiences can be profoundly healing, and often enable the person to let go and die at peace.

Dying process involves changes to circulation to brain and this can cause hallucinatory changes. These include dying person to speak of being visited by dead relatives, moving in and out of reality, and describe other-worldly realms. They may speak of embarking on a journey, or may suddenly stare at a point in the room or turn towards the window and experience a sense of amazement, joy or wonder. They may also appear to be thinking deeply, as if they are being 'shown' information that they may not have considered before. Dying people, and those who witness these end of life experiences, usually describe them with loving, reassuring words such as calming, soothing, greeting, comforting, beautiful, readying. It is not known how many dying people have such visions and experiences, but research suggests that end of life visions and dreams hold profound meaning for dying people, helping them to come to terms with their dying process.

END OF LIFE CARE

The goal of care for people who are dying focuses on helping them enjoy as good a quality of life as possible. This may include relieving suffering and pain, helping people stay as well as they can and helping them achieve goals that are important to them before they die. This care is often provided by a mix of professionals, including those skilled in palliative care. These professionals will want to ensure that everyone affected by a terminal condition knows about the choices they have and what support is available to them at this difficult time.

Some people are fortunate in being able to approach their dying process at peace with themselves and with those they love. But that's not always the case. People can be frightened, confused, unable to express what they're feeling or what they need. Person may be afraid to die and may feel he is a burden to their friends, family or society. He may be angry and feel cheated. Some may feel lost and alone, and desperate for someone to ask how they truly feel. They may feel angry and let down by their belief. They may be clinging onto hope for a miracle cure. They may feel as if they have wasted their life and are grieving missed opportunities. They may be desperate to die. They may want to make contact with ex-partners or estranged family or friends. They may want to confess to things that have happened in the past, or to ask for forgiveness. This can be painful and upsetting for relatives, but it can also be powerfully healing. They may also become irrationally angry and resentful. They may be missing relatives and friends who are unable to be with them. It is important to realise the behaviour of a dying person is not always rational.

If you caring for someone with terminal illness, you need to put your own life on hold. when someone is dying you will probably find it impossible to do or to think of anything else apart from being with them or preparing for their death. And when you are not with them, you will be on red alert and thinking about them. You may feel as if you are unable to focus, and to relate to normal life. Everyday conversations may seem trivial and irrelevant. Explain clearly to your employers and family members what you are going through. Additional stresses and strains can feel hard to bear. Some dying people may want to see friends and extended family, but others may not. This can change from day to day. Always check with them before inviting people to visit. Nearer the end, it may be okay to offer people the opportunity to come and say their farewells. Some will gladly do this. Others may not, preferring to remember the dying person as they were.

To alleviate discomfort, a dying person may be attached to medical equipment such as a syringe-driver, monitors and a respirator. This can be alarming for relatives and friends to begin with. It's also hard to be with someone who is semi-conscious, in physical or emotional distress, and who may be moaning or crying out. You may yourself feel very anxious and helpless, and at times, overwhelmed, vulnerable and lonely, especially when nursing staff are busy with other patients. Make sure you take plenty of breaks, although it can be hard to find a private place when things get tough. But there are often quiet rooms in hospices, and hospital chapels are usually open around the clock. You may feel guilty when you go home knowing you might never see the person again. That's normal. Just make sure when you leave you say your goodbyes. These farewells can mount up as the days go by.

A death in the family, especially when it's the last parent, can throw up a lot of unresolved and painful issues. Some members of the family will have had a warm relationship with the dying person. Others may be harboring dislike, grudges or anger. Some will freely embrace what is happening. Others may want to deny that the person is dying. Some will be happy to stop life-extending treatment. Others may not want this. Some may feel horrified by the person's deterioration and find it difficult to sit with them. Relatives who live at a distance may feel guilty for not being there. Others may avoid contact due to family conflict. Relatives who care for the dying person may feel their own life is on hold and become angry and resentful with the rest of the family if they feel they are not pulling their weight. Sibling rivalry may surface and divide loyalties, causing further resentments and disputes. Some relatives may be privy to secrets that no-one else knows, and find this distressing. So, be prepared for this to be an intensely emotional time which needs patience, understanding and a willingness to communicate openly and truthfully with the rest of the family. Sadly, this is not always possible, and disputes can happen or deepen.

REACTING TO A DEATH

At some point in our lives though, we are likely to have to deal with the death of other people who are close to us. This may require some further thinking, but the perspective we have gained in relation to our own lives (and deaths) will help us here too.

First, Accept the possibility of it. It is of course a major shock when anyone close to you dies, but at least don't let the possibility that they could die in the first place be a shock to you. What I mean by this is that, by having an acceptance of the possibility of the death of those we love at the back of our minds at all times, we can not only remind ourselves to make the best of these relationships while they're there, but also make it slightly easier to come to terms with these events if they happen. Even considering this possibility can be a difficult thing to do, especially with our children or partners. This doesn't however have to take the form of a morbid obsession with the impending doom of our loved ones, but rather an acceptance of it as a reality of being alive, of the fragility of life and of having emotional connections to other people.

Appreciate the relationships you have. A parallel point to some of those made in part one of this booklet, we can use our acceptance of the reality of death, and the brevity of life (including of those we love) to remind us to make the most of our relationships and the time spent with people we love. In short, we should use our perspective on death to enhance our appreciation of life. Don't feel bad about how you react. We all react differently to major life events, so the last thing you need to do during the testing time of dealing with the death of someone close to you is to judge yourself on how you're reacting compared to others and worry about whether it's the 'right' reaction. Let them go, If you are close to someone who is dying or whose life is threatened, challenge yourself to check that you are making decisions and giving advice that is based on what is best for the person and what they want – rather than what you want. That's why it is so beneficial when people make their wishes known before, they are dying.

When we face the threat of losing someone we love, it can be extremely difficult to step back from our overwhelming desire to preserve their life and keep them around us, but try to make sure that you are thinking about it from their perspective. Try to look to the future, being told of the need to 'move on' after a bereavement might seem to be a very cold and unrealistic idea, which completely fails to understand how the bereaved person may be feeling. Despite this though, there seems to be some value in trying to accept the transience of things, even ourselves and the people we love the most, and using this to stop us holding on to anything too much, both people and anything else in life. This idea, used by Buddhism and several other schools of thought, can be very hard to follow as most of us cling to things in life, often quite naturally, as these things can give our lives meaning. Perhaps though, it could help us to see other people as gifts that come into our lives that we don't own and can't hold on to forever. This in turn might make it a little easier to try to continue our lives making new attachments rather than letting the loss of past ones make our lives unbearable.

SUMMARY

Line between providing a cure and taking good care of an ill person is thin but clearly demarcated. However, it is beneficial for the care of the person to demarcate it clearly. Honesty and kindness should be balanced. Persons choice should be paramount important. Where a person is incapable of expressing his own wishes, the best interest option should be adopted.

NO SURPRISE

Dear death, we never met, I don't know you,

And I know, what I don't know, can't hurt you.

No surprises, when we meet, I will wait and be alert,

Once we meet, I won't exist, so still I won't be hurt.

My body served my "self" all along

Now I have no self, it is time, I could not prolong,

I salute the nature and the elements of the earth,

Here I come to join you, and to become a part.

Scatter my ashes where gentle winds blow,

Let it go far and fall where the paddy plants grow.

From the strength of the ashes, if a crop spring,

Fulfilled will be my gratitude in life, I sing.

9 WHAT HAPPENS WHEN I DIE

Death is not a metaphysical mysterious event. For ages, death involved tap on the shoulder from Grim Reaper or noose from the agent of Yama around your neck. Now we know different. Death is a biological, physiological event resulting in loss of biological and physiological functions, with end, resulting in a physical, mechanical remains.

LAST STAGES OF LIFE

Many physical changes occur during the process of dying that affect the emotional, social, and spiritual aspects of a person's life. Health professionals speak of "dying trajectories" that suggest how persons with specific diseases will die. For example, those with a terminal illness, such as advanced cancer, will show a steady decline toward death. Those with serious chronic illnesses may have highs and lows that sometimes give the impression of recovery.

Remember that each person's death is unique. In the final stages of a terminal illness, it can become evident that in spite of the best care, attention, and treatment, you are approaching the end of life. At this point, the focus usually changes to making you as comfortable as possible in order to make the most of the time you have left. Depending on the nature of the illness and your circumstances, this final stage period may last from a matter of weeks or months to several years. During this time, palliative care measures can help to control pain and other symptoms, such as constipation, nausea, or shortness of breath. Hospice care can also offer emotional and spiritual support to both the patient and their family.

It is helpful to understand the common symptoms experienced in people who are dying. You may observe none, some, or all of these symptoms in the dying person's last days and hours on earth. You will also learn things to do that can help ease physical pain and suffering. As the end of life approaches, there is a feeling of detachment from the physical world and a loss of interest in things formerly found pleasurable. There is a tendency to sleep more. There is less desire to talk. This is the beginning of letting go of life and preparing for death. Days or hours before death, the dying person becomes less and less responsive to voice and touch and may not awaken. Sometimes, quite unexpectedly, the person may appear well and even look as if he is going to recover.

Visual or auditory hallucinations are often part of the dying experience. The appearance of family members or loved ones who have died is common. These visions are considered normal. The dying may turn their focus to "another world" and talk to people or see things that others do not see. This can be unsettling, but purely hallucinatory.

As death nears, the dying person may lose interest in food and drink. The ability to swallow becomes impaired. Loss of appetite and reduced intake are normal parts of dying. In the early stages of dying, the dying person may prefer only soft foods and liquids. In the very last stages of life, however, they may not want any food or drink. A dying person may want to suck on ice chips or take a small amount of liquid, just to wet and freshen the mouth, which can become very dry. Forcing fluid may cause choking, or the dying person may draw liquid into the lungs, making matters worse.

It is hard for most people to respect the dying person's lack of appetite. That's because many of us equate food with caring. Family members may feel that withholding nutrition is cruel or neglectful. They may worry that they are starving their loved one. It is important to remember that as the physical body is dying, the vital organs are shutting down, and nourishment is no longer required to keep them functioning.

The two major concerns are constipation and incontinence (loss of control over bowel and bladder functions). Constipation may be caused by lack of mobility, pain medication, and decreased fluid intake. Laxatives are generally needed to keep the bowels clean. Incontinence, or loss of bowel and bladder control, is likely to be distressing to the dying person and those in attendance. As death nears, the muscles in these areas relax further and contents are released.

Restlessness and agitation are common. These symptoms may be caused by reduced oxygen to the brain, metabolic changes, dehydration, and pain medications. "Terminal delirium" is a condition that may be seen when the person is very close to death, marked by extreme restlessness and agitation. Although it may look distressing, this condition is not considered to be painful.

There are medications available to control symptoms. Be aware there may be unfinished business. Dying persons may try to hold on until they feel a sense of security and completion. Picking, pulling, and fidgeting behaviours may also be seen. This can result from medications, metabolic changes, or decreased oxygen to the brain.

You may observe that breathing is shallow and quickened, or slow and contrived. The person may make gurgling sounds, sometimes referred to as the "death rattle." These sounds are due to the pooling of secretions and an inability to cough them up. The air passing through the mucus causes this sound. The breathing pattern most disturbing to witnesses, called Cheyne-Stokes breathing, is marked by periods of no breathing at all (up to 45 seconds), followed by deeper and more frequent respirations. These respirations are common and result from decreased oxygen supply to the vital organs and a build-up of waste products in the body.

As death nears, it's very common for a person's breathing to change, sometimes slowing, other times speeding up or becoming noisy and shallow. The changes are triggered by reduction in blood flow, and they're not painful.

This condition is not uncomfortable or painful for the dying person, although it may be unsettling to observe. The "death rattle" or Cheyne-Stokes breathing indicate that death is near. As the body dies, the blood moves away from the extremities toward the vital organs. You may notice that while the extremities are cool, the abdomen is warm. You may notice changes in body temperature.

Instead of simply sleeping more, the person's consciousness may begin to fluctuate, making them nearly impossible to wake at times, even when there is a lot of stimulation around them.

The dying person may feel hot one minute and cold the next. As death approaches, there may be high fever. You also may see purplish-bluish blotches and mottling on the legs, arms or on the underside of the body where blood may be collecting. As death nears, the body may appear yellowish or waxen in colour. Most physical pain can be controlled. No one should die in pain when the means to relieve it are available. All persons have the right to have their pain controlled.

Pain is real. Always believe a person who says he/she has pain. Remember that each person is an individual and perceptions of pain differ. Managing pain and discomfort requires daily monitoring and reassessment of your loved one's subtle nonverbal signals. Slight behavioural changes can indicate their needs aren't being met. Communicating such changes to your loved one's medical team will provide valuable clues about their level of pain. You can also help to ease your loved one's discomfort through touch, massage, music, fragrance, and the sound of your soothing voice. Experiment with different approaches and observe your loved one's reactions.

There are certain signs in the last few weeks, days and sometimes hours of life that indicate when someone is preparing to die. Recognising what these are will help you to say those important goodbyes, and prepare yourself for what is to come.

The point of no return, when a person begins deteriorating towards their final breath, can start weeks or months before someone dies. Simple actions, such as going from a bed to a chair, can become exhausting. A dying person often starts to withdraw from the news, some activities and other people, to talk less or have trouble with conversation, and to sleep more. This all ties in with a drop in energy levels caused by a deterioration in the body's brain function and metabolic processes.

Predicting exactly when a person will die is, of course, nearly impossible and depends on factors ranging from the health issues they have to whether they are choosing to accept more medical interventions. As the body continues to wind down, various other reflexes and functions will also slow. A dying person will become progressively more fatigued, their sleep-wake patterns more random, their coughing and swallowing reflexes slower. They will start to respond less to verbal commands and gentle touch. Reduced blood flow to the brain or chemical imbalances can also cause a dying person to become disoriented, confused or detached from reality and time. Visions or hallucinations often come into play.

With the slowing in blood circulation, body temperature can begin to seesaw, so a person can be cool to the touch at one point and then hot later on.

An irregular breathing pattern known as Cheyne-Stokes is also often seen in people approaching death: taking one or several breaths followed by a long pause with no breathing at all, then another breath. Gradually, the person drifts in and out or slips into complete unconsciousness.

PROCESS OF DEATH

'The stoppage of circulation, the inadequate transport of oxygen to tissue, the flickering out of brain function, the failure of organs, the destruction of vital centres- these are the weapons of every horseman of death'. Nature has a job to do. It does its job by the method that seems most suited to each individual. (Sherwin Nuland in *"How we die"*). Everyone wants to know details of death and dying. That is human nature. We are irresistibly attracted to dangers affecting our life. It is easy to summarise the various ways a human can die in medical terms. That would be description of the cessation of the functioning of the body. But the human death is more than that. There are three distinct entities which make up an alive human being.

First entity is the body, the identity of life is carried by the body in a distinct recognisable shape and persona. Formation of the body starts from the moment of fertilisation of the egg. Carefully orchestrated events of embryogenesis guided by decoding of the genetic information results in growth and formation of the organs. Slowly throughout young age body maturation attains full adult function. Many human adult activities focus around looking after the body, keeping it in ideal shape, condition and disease free.

Second is the intellect, the cognitive functions and behaviour characteristic of the individual. Cognitive functions are the mental processes or brain functions that allow us to receive, select, store, transform, develop, and recover information. Individuals have unique way of processing the external stimulus. This forms their characteristic. Cognitive functioning refers to multiple mental abilities, including learning, thinking, reasoning, remembering, problem solving, decision making, and attention. Over the period of lifespan, individuals gather vast amount of information, develop knowledge and skills, which are retained and developed throughout the life.

Third a biological process which allows the body to function and carry out the cognitive functions. Physiological processes of assimilation of nutrition, absorption and distribution of oxygen, elimination of metabolic waste and maintaining constant internal environment facilitate functioning of the body and brain. There is no life in the body without underlying biological supportive process nor there be any cognitive functions.

When death occurs, all three elements cease to function. The biological process of respiration, homeostasis and circulation stop. This results in degradation of the cells hence putrefaction of the body. Absence of the physical body and biological process to sustain it, will immediately result in loss of progressive changes in persons cognitive and mental capacity. Though some automated parts of the individual's identity, economic assets and intellectual works may appear to remain in memory of other people or in digital media, they become static and uninfluenced further by the person.

Notably there is no element which continues to leave the body upon occurrence of death, and certainly nothing what needs to be reunited with supernatural powers. Perhaps the soul constitutes of the biological process sustaining life of the body and the intellectual cognitive characteristic of the individual. Both of these will peacefully cease to exist upon death. Hence all the ceremonial and religious treatment of death becomes rather unnecessary. Decline in each of these entities is part of dying process. However, the term death is generally used to describe complete cessation of all three occurring as singular event.

Dying process is not horror filled degradation, but it is disintegration of human life. There is not much dignity about it specially for the family involved. The greatest dignity to find in death is the dignity of life preceded it. We seek the ways to mask the images of death from everywhere. Most deaths in modern society happen in hospitals or hospice care homes. It may appear the death is hidden, sanitised and packaged neatly to burial, but it does not reduce the importance of being aware and prepared.

We can't generalise the dying process. The process of dying varies depending on the cause. Also depending on which definition of death you follow; the timing of death may be variable. First concept, we need to understand is that, death, in all elements does not occur in a singular event. There are multiple physiologic systems interdependent on each other in the body. If one slows down the other try to compensate, but if one shut down or severely compromised, other systems can't keep functioning for long, and they turn off slowly. So, depending on what system slows down first, the death process unravels in a sequence. Second concept, even after measurable parameters, like electrocardiogram, or electrical brainwave, or body temperature, pulse, breathing cease to show, there still remains some biochemical changes in the cellular and chemical levels. And this can continue for long time after clinical death. Third concept, some organs in the body can function longer than others and will be able to revive with active support than the others. We can stimulate breathing, restart a heart which has stopped beating after several minutes but we can't repair the damage to the brain once it sets in.

In case of blood loss in a traumatic incident, or a circulatory collapse due to septic shock, or severe allergic reaction, it is the circulation of blood which collapses first. This produces inadequate perfusion to the brain and vital tissue, thereby causing brain death, cardiac arrest etc. ultimately causing death. In case of a myocardial infarction or heart attack, the output of blood pumping suffers first, causing circulation failure, this again follows the path of a circulatory collapse.

I case of a drowning, or smoke inhalation or lung inflammation like pneumonia, it is the oxygenation of blood which is affected first. Even though circulation is adequate, blood is not adequately oxygenated, thereby causing tissue damage in vital organs causing death.

In specific organ failures like liver and kidney, specific functions of the organs deteriorate causing internal derangement of acidity, enzymes and ionic concentration in blood. Tissues like brain is very sensitive to these changes and cease to function at certain level of changes causing control failure on vital organs.

I recognise medically dying process is neither as simple as I have tried to explain, nor there is asset pattern of changes in every pathology. But examples will help to stress on the concepts I have discussed.

DIMINISHING CONCIOUSNESS

Most deaths are preceded by diminishing level of consciousness. Is this beneficial? There are several beliefs and phenomena associated with diminishing brain capacity nearing death. I feel it is appropriate to address the issues in brief.

Reducing blood supply to brain is an age-related change. This results in reduced cognitive function, onset of dementia and inability to coordinate certain neuromuscular activity. However nearing death, the deterioration of brain function is rapid. This results in loss of sense of self. Loss of frontal cortical activity, I feel is a defensive mechanism by evolution, protecting the person against gloom of impending death. This will terminate thought process and perhaps shield against pain and anxiety in the process of dying. This intern can reduce stress hormone and chemical induced pain, anxiety and behavioural changes in the dying person. In very crude wording, you don't remain sane enough to go insane!

Some part of the brain will still retain function and some blood supply. The reducing blood supply to parts of the brain can cause tunnel vison and other visual and auditory hallucinations. Some of these feelings have been described as near-death experience phenomena, such as life events flashing, floating around, or seeing dead relatives. These hallucinatory effects have contributed to many death related beliefs.

People with lower level of consciousness can still hear and sometime can respond to stimulus. Person have still had memories and feeling of touch and hearing stimulus. It is therefore important to provide care and peace to the dying person in the last moment. Sometimes moderate renewal of blood flow or energy release may make person to show brief signs of regaining consciousness. This is not a sign of recovery and lasts very short period. It is also known that due to this phenomenon, some people gain enough consciousness to be able to speak briefly before dying.

CELLULAR AND BODY CHANGES AFTER DEATH

Decomposition begins several minutes after death with a process called autolysis, or self-digestion. Soon after the heart stops beating, cells become deprived of oxygen, and their acidity increases as the toxic by-products of chemical reactions begin to accumulate inside them. Enzymes start to digest cell membranes and then leak out as the cells break down. This usually begins in the liver, which is rich in enzymes, and in the brain, which has high water content. Eventually, though, all other tissues and organs begin to break down in this way. Damaged blood cells begin to spill out of broken vessels and, aided by gravity, settle in the capillaries and small veins, discolouring the skin.

Body temperature also begins to drop, until it has acclimatised to its surroundings. Then, rigor mortis – "the stiffness of death" – sets in, starting in the eyelids, jaw and neck muscles, before working its way into the trunk and then the limbs. In life, muscle cells contract and relax due to the actions of two filamentous proteins (actin and myosin), which slide along each other. After death, the cells are depleted of their energy source and the protein filaments become locked in place. This causes the muscles to become rigid and locks the joints.

During these early stages, the cadaveric ecosystem consists mostly of the bacteria that live in and on the living human body. Our bodies host huge numbers of bacteria; every one of the body's surfaces and corners provides a habitat for a specialised microbial community. By far the largest of these communities resides in the gut, which is home to trillions of bacteria of hundreds or perhaps thousands of different species.

The gut microbiome has been linked to roles in human health and a plethora of conditions and diseases, from autism and depression to irritable bowel syndrome and obesity. But we still know little about these microbial passengers while we are alive. We know even less about what happens to them when we die. Most internal organs are devoid of microbes when we are alive. Soon after death, however, the immune system stops working, leaving them to spread throughout the body freely. This usually begins in the gut, at the junction between the small and large intestines. Left unchecked, our gut bacteria begin to digest the intestines – and then the surrounding tissues – from the inside out, using the chemical cocktail that leaks out of damaged cells as a food source. Then they invade the capillaries of the digestive system and lymph nodes, spreading first to the liver and spleen, then into the heart and brain.

Once self-digestion is under way and bacteria have started to escape from the gastrointestinal tract, putrefaction begins. This is molecular death – the breakdown of soft tissues even further, into gases, liquids and salts. It is already under way at the earlier stages of decomposition but really gets going when anaerobic bacteria get in on the act.

Putrefaction is associated with a marked shift from aerobic bacterial species, which require oxygen to grow, to anaerobic ones, which do not. These then feed on the body's tissues, fermenting the sugars in them to produce gaseous by-products such as methane, hydrogen sulphide and ammonia, which accumulate within the body, inflating or 'bloating' the abdomen and sometimes other body parts.

This causes further discolouration of the body. As damaged blood cells continue to leak from disintegrating vessels, anaerobic bacteria convert haemoglobin molecules, which once carried oxygen around the body, into sulfhaemoglobin. The presence of this molecule in settled blood gives skin the marbled, greenish-black appearance characteristic of a body undergoing active decomposition. An average human body consists of 50–75% water, and every kilogram of dry body mass eventually releases 32g of nitrogen, 10g of phosphorous, 4g of potassium and 1g of magnesium into the soil.

DIPOSAL OF PHYSICAL REMAINS

Disposal of the dead is a significant activity affecting personal, emotional, social and environmental matters. As the population in the world is increasing, the disposal methods need to adapt to most environmentally friendly and least space consuming. Disposal of the physical remains is a sensitive yet inevitable and essential activity. Key environmental concerns include land use, land space of the graveyards and pollution implications.

Burial as a means of removing the dead is an ancient practice. Where burials are influenced by Islamic and Jewish faiths, preparation involves the washing of the corpse and containment in a wooden coffin. In China, traditional preference is to use methods of disposal to delay the decay, by packing the coffin with clothing and shrouds. Embalming, though not traditional, is practiced in Europe and north America, for preservation of the body. Process of burial affect the land and can prevent the use of the land for future. Cemeteries have capacity constraints, mainly in urban areas. They require regular maintenance. Land is a finite resource, and large and expanding cemetery usage may conflict with farming, residential, industrial and leisure activities.

Traditional Indian cultural belief in many religions is that the human body and the universe is made of five elements, air, water, fire, earth and space. The last rites of passage are to return the human body to the elements of the nature, to its origin. Various methods of ceremonial disposal are practiced on this Vedic principle. The use of cremation for disposing the physical remains is common practice in countries influenced by Hindu and Sikh faiths. There are environmental consequences for cremation, in terms of energy consumption and emissions. Of particular concern in many countries, is the release of mercury from dental amalgam resulting from cremation. Mongolian culture is famous, along with the Vajrayana Buddhist from Tibet, which leaves the body of the deceased on a high unprotected place to be exposed to the elements and devoured by wildlife. It is part of the Buddhist thinking that body after death need not be respected. This type of sky burial is also practiced in other cultures.

Scattering of the ashes is a universal practice which has caused significant environmental concerns. Pollution of river Ganges, fear of contaminating lake Constance for example. Alternative natural burial such as sea burial are relatively environmentally less damaging and should be preferred. Use of biodegradable coffins and shroud materials could be looked at.

For all of us, to make that small step, towards helping the environment, the ability to choose a banana leaf or a cardboard cask instead of a metal and wood coffin, a body without embalming for quick degradation, should give a sense of control. Use of sustainable materials which does not use huge amount of energy and low emissions should make you feel better about what your choices are for the earth you are leaving behind. Where religious practices do not dominate, the natural burial with ecological concerns should be promoted. The future may offer more choices that reduce the impact on land usage and pollution. Research is underway to convert bodies into liquid or freeze-dried granular fertiliser.

One day, cemeteries, with rich nutrients coming from decomposing bodies can become gardens and orchards of lush food plants. Fertilized by all that nitrogen, phosphorus, potash, trace elements and organic matter that dead bodies would provide, cemeteries become lush gardens of fruits, grains, vegetables, and trees for food and for building materials with a farmer's market at the entrance to sell the produce. Tombstones could be shaped like benches for visitors to rest from weeding their cemetery garden plots, or from pruning their cemetery trees, or just to relax while eating lunch or engaging in idle conversation.

SUMMARY

End of life is no a metaphysical event. It is ending of a biological process resulting in a non-living corpse from a living individual. The process may start dignified, but it is process involving termination of life. It can be distressing but need not involve pain. It may emotional but with right preparation, we can reduce the despair.

Pinnacle of Life

ME AND MY SOUL

I am bit confused, how I came to be a being?

if someone created me, am I part of that thing?

I know who I am, from beginning to the end,

all this talk of spirit and soul, I can't comprehend.

I have a brain, I have a mind and I can think and dream,

never did work with spirit or soul, together as a team.

If we are living in the same body, without any qualm

My soul must be gentle, friendly and full of real charm.

I wanted to search inside my body, for my mate, my soul,

Heart, lungs, top to toe I scroll, not a sign of this enigmatic black hole.

Alas, we depart, when I rest in peace, we would go apart,

Whatever you become, wish you very best, from bottom of my heart.

Pinnacle of Life

10 FACING BEREAVEMENT

As death is universal, so are the acts that follow it. Disposal of physical remains, grief or grieving, funeral, mourning and other cultural and religious events follow any death. There is no particular order and the actual process and events vary in every culture and religion. Even in a society with same religion and culture, the rituals may be different and very unique. But the theme seems to be universal. Funeral rituals have evolved in response to the loss in the society caused by death, and the perceived threat from it. Funeral and burial rites vary significantly across cultures, and are influenced by each culture's conceptions of death and dying. The rituals change the identity of the person from living to dead. The new identity may be as a memory or a photograph on the wall, spirit of an ancestor, a preserved corpse, or a soul that returns to its origin.

The rituals practiced in may religions focus on preparing the dead to migrate to another world. Depending on the nature of belief, either the spirit or the soul is released, or helped to migrate to another world or become on with spiritual powers. Example the Hindu "Shraaddha" ceremony, held on the twelfth day after death marks the end of the mourning, allows the soul to leave the dead permanently and go to a better place. Lengthy chants and generous gifts ensure the process goes smoothly.

I feel the whole process is focused on preparing the soul of the dead rather than addressing mental and emotional wellbeing of the living relatives. There is little time to worry about the bereaved Family. That needs to change. Celebration of the life of dead person, family gathering, expression of social bonds and solidarity are positive aspects of these events, but these can be done in more relaxed and less prescriptive way. Example, the ceremony does not need to be on a fixed day, rather a more convenient day, allow everyone to travel and be present, no one need to miss it because it is prescribed date by an unknown scripture.

FACING BEREAVEMENT.

Death of a person may be an end of all his presence - physical, spiritual, digital, intellectual and many other ways. All forms human connection with other human beings comes to an end. This way, bereavement affects the living more than what effect it has on the person who has died. The trauma of thought not able to see someone you lived with for long time, someone you cared for, someone whom you would turn to in the time of difficulty is hard to overcome. This is where the real grief and tragedy of death strikes. The feeling of emptiness and vacuum in the space occupied by the person diseased can be overwhelming. Yet filling that space with religious and cultural beliefs which are bare psychological management of mind is not justifiable.

"Tell your friend, when he dies, a bit of you will die too. The bit, which is your friendship, will be no more. That way nobody dies alone"

We have a good understanding of functioning of our mind. Society is strong enough to face the reality of a bereavement. More is needed in this field in the form of education and involvement of social institutions to support the bereaved families. It is the true memory of the person, the memories which would stay with you for ever makes the person immortal, not the shrines and offerings.

Pinnacle of Life

There is positive in every death. A lesson. An opportunity. A change of guard. When a death occurs, there are three practical elements face the family and friends.

First, sense of loss, grief of not seeing someone any longer. However, death is natural, unfathomable and inevitable. Death can potentially relieve the person from human sufferings, pain, illness and anxiety. Grieving should be about coming to terms with the loss, remembering the passion and principles the person lived her life, and not dictated by compulsive acts of ceremonious offerings and chants.

Second, the space occupied by the person in day to day life. Perhaps as someone made family meals, or person who opened the door when bell rings or the head of the family and the executor of the family business. Not matter what role the person played; they will be dearly missed. Same applies outside the house, social place or work place. There are two distinct elements to overcoming the void created by the loss of a person. Death of a person creates a void and someone, or collectively many, need to step up to fill the void. And there is effect of time, passing of time makes the roughness of the loss feel smoother.

Third, and most difficult event is degree of confusion by the loss. Inability to understand the wishes of the dead person and what they would have liked you to do. Bereaved families and friends also go through stages from denial to acceptance. Grief can begin before a loved one has died, and this anticipatory grief helps lessen later distress. During the next stage of grief, after the death of the loved one, mourners are likely to cry, have trouble sleeping, and lose their appetite. Some feel alarmed, angry, or wounded by being left behind. After formal services for the deceased are over and conventional forms of social support end, depression and loneliness often occur.

Feelings of guilt are quite common, and in some individuals think seriously about taking their own life for somehow failing the loved one. This is especially true in response to the loss of a child. Though people often talk about healthy and unhealthy grief, it is very difficult to measure emotional pain way or advise how long one's grief should last. Many clinicians believe that those who abandon their grief prematurely are living in denial and make healing more difficult. But, on the other hand, it is also possible to become over involved in despair.

GRIEF AND BREAVEMENT

Grief is combination of several different emotions which are expressed at the time death of a significant other person. Grief, bereavement, and mourning are common terms which are repeatedly used in the literature. In an attempt to define one term, many authors employ the other terms due to their interdependence. Regardless of their extensive use, no words can fully explain profound meaning grief. Events leading to death such as terminal illness do not end with the death of the dying person. In fact, all humans, including the dying, experience grief as a response to impeding or resultant death. Grief is a personal emotional reaction. Bereavement refers to the experiences that follow the death of a loved one, while mourning is the process through which grief is expressed. Mourning thus represents the culturally accepted expression of the personal feelings that follow the death.

Bereavement is the state of having suffered a loss or is a state caused by loss. Bereavement is an umbrella term that describes the events and consequences that take place after the loss. Several types of losses can create the state of bereavement. The term bereavement has roots in the old English language and means "to rob," "to plunder," or "to dispossess". It also has the idea of taking away a loved one in a forceful manner leaving the survivor struggling with the experience of a sudden loss and separation. Bereavement like phenomenon has been described in groups who made sudden life changes like immigration and job loss.

Mourning has been referred to as the external expression. It is like any other emotional expression, is socially regulated. It is the outer manifestation and public demonstration of grief. Mourning is bereavement shared publicly. It is the act of lamenting openly the lost object or deceased person. The term mourning could have two meanings. The first is derived from the psychoanalytic literature and implies a wide range of conscious and unconscious activities and intrapsychic processes, all triggered by the event of loss. The second refers to the appropriate cultural response to grief over a major loss.

My father died after a short illness, at home. I was 24 and was studying for my master's degree. I knew very little about the death, dying and bereavement process. I can outline what I recall. I was with my father to give him the Ganges water as a last rite. The after-death events were a proper family and community affair with religious guidance. Hindu tradition dictates that the body be washed and prepared for cremation, as a process of cleanliness. There are no funeral directors, the guidance is provided by the elderly. There was no hearse or coffin, the body was carried on a traditional make shift stretcher on the shoulder by the relatives and well wishers. There was no embalming, the cremation was carried out withing few hours after death. It is a traditional belief in Hindu culture, that the dead body is an unnecessary weight burden on mother earth, and should be disposed without delay. I did not pay anyone for any of the services, everyone pulled together in a community spirit and out of respect to my father except for the specialist priest. There were herbs, sandal wood garlands, clarified butter and flowers. There was huge gathering at the cremation ground, my relatives, my father's colleagues and students. There was no intimation or invitation, people had turned up on their own accord. The mourning period was somewhat dictated by the events of lengthy rituals and ceremonies. There was expression of grief. I took consolation by the remarks the priest made in the end, that I had done everything as expected. Gifts were made to charities and brahmin priests. I still vividly remember everyone who came to help me that day, with a sense of gratitude. I feel the social gathering reinforced the bonds. It is at the time of crisis that the great strengths of the community appear. The support and help prove of great value.

Would I have done anything differently? Yes. Admittedly my father died at an age lower than the average life expectancy. He was terminally ill for some time. But we were thoroughly unprepared. We all knew of his impending death. But we never spoke about it. There was no death awareness. No thoughts, no dialogue. He Often spoke to me about my life after his death, but never about his own death. Should I have had a discussion, it would have made my grieving process so much easier. Similar thoughts must have affected all the members of my family, at that time, and ever since. Being death aware and death prepared, not only takes the weight of the shoulders of the dying person, but also reduces the anxiety of the loved one's. As the events of COVID-19 have shown, tomorrow is not the time, the dialogue can start today. I regret spending too much time on the religious prescription, of various symbolic rituals. I should have focused more on emotional wellbeing of the family, and the grieving and myself.

EVOLUTION OF GRIEF

Grief, after death of someone may be profound because it, reminds us of our own mortality. It is also modulated by the stress hormones secreted as a result of anxiety, which could again be related to underlying thought about our own loss. Evolutionary biologists think that grief is passed as a side effect of having relationships. Biological reaction to separation keeps us together because staying together provides an evolutionary benefit. Humans are primarily group animals, and living together has survival benefits. Like in children and parents, relationship evolutionarily, rely on one another for protection. In more social animals, such as humans, those reciprocal relationships extend beyond parent-child. "Grief, in its most basic form, represents an alarm reaction set off by a deficit signal in the behavioural system underlying attachment,".

There is clear lack of research in grief, same is lack of thinking about death. Grief like death is not the favourite subject of investigation by scientists including psychologists. While there is a large science and knowledge regarding pathological aspect of grief and its management, there is little acceptance of study of normal grief process.

Grief following loss of a person happens in stages. Many stages have been described include shock, disorganization, volatile emotions, sense of loss, loneliness, relief and re-establishment. David Fulcomer described four distinct stage of grief reaction. The immediate stage, includes stoic, dazed, collapse, and emotional response like crying. The post immediate stage included protest, detachment, attention gathering, and excitement. The transitional stage to re-entry to active life, and the final stage of memory phantasy and repression.

There is a wide variation across cultures in how people behave after a death and how they are expected to behave. Regardless of the specific ways in which the grief process is manifested, it is postulated to involve many themes and issues that people invariably confront. In some cultures, close relatives are expected to shave their heads, wear either white or black clothing, and express grief for a specified minimum period of time. In other cultures, mourning involves a lot of drinking, dancing, and in some cases, a person within a certain position is expected to marry the spouse of the deceased. In yet other cultures, the requirements for dealing with a major loss are played out over the balance of the lifetime of the survivor. This could be in form of rituals, what is worn, how one is to be addressed by others, and one's rights and obligations to participate in various activities within the community.

GRIEF REACTIONS

The most common reactions are, sense of shock and disbelief, numbness, substantial sadness, irritation and anger, guilt and self-reproach. Various symptoms of anxiety, including shortness of breath, hollowness in the stomach, and tightness in the throat, all sorts of fears and apprehensions may develop. Intense yearning, crying, tearfulness, and sobbing, sorrowfulness, deep frustration sleep and appetite disturbances are common. These reactions may occur in or out of sequence, mixed or combined, separate or together. Some of them are short and intermittent in nature while others persist for a long period of time. Typically, what makes a loss especially devastating is its magnitude, finality, and irreversibility.

Two integrative approaches have been proposed to more

specifically enhance the understanding of how people process grief. These are the four-component and the dual process models of grief and bereavement. The four-component model, which is based largely on emotion theory and has some commonalities with the transactional model of stress, suggests that four things are needed in order to understand grief. The first is the context in which the loss occurred – death could be expected or unexpected; sudden or gradual. The second is the continuum of meaning associated with the loss. This could range from examining what one may do on an everyday basis to reflecting on the long-term and substantial issues of what the loss entails. The third issue deals with changing the representations of the lost relationship over time. As time passes, the survivor may begin to modify their previous roles and begin to adapt to new ways of functioning. The fourth is the part that coping and emotion regulation processes play in all coping strategies that survivor uses in dealing with grief. These issues involved in the four-component model clearly indicate that processing grief is complicated and its outcome is often unclear, and becomes evident only after some passage of time.

The dual process model is also an integrative approach because it incorporates existing ideas concerning stressors. The dual-process model identifies two major types of stressors: Loss-oriented stressors that are associated with the loss itself such as breaking ties with the deceased and grief work that has to be undertaken. Restoration oriented stressors are those associated with adapting to new life situations, this might include adopting new roles or identities, including new relationships, and finding distractions from grief. The dual process model suggests that dealing with these stressors tends to require a dynamic process that involves the survivor constantly and interchangeably engaged in both dealing with the grief and efforts to adapt to a new life without the deceased.

When a bereaved person expresses intense feelings of loneliness, guilt, and overwhelmingly focuses on the loss to the point where it interferes with their everyday functioning, they are said to have prolonged grief disorder, a condition that is distinguishable from depression.

FUNERAL AND BURIAL RITUALS

Death is the final life transition. The funeral is often considered as a celebration of a rite of passage for both the deceased and the living. Societies tend to surround death with specific rituals that are aimed at assisting the bereaved through this final life transition. Funeral rites are believed to serve three closely intertwined functions. When a member of a society dies, there arises a need to realign the relationships among the survivors. The first function of the funeral is obviously to dispose of the body of the deceased. Funerals also serve psychological and social purposes among which include: to explain, justify, and regulate the new social relationships that are created by the death. Additionally, the funeral is part of a longer ritual that takes the dead safely out of this world and into the next. After the funeral rituals are concluded, the immediate family may practice other rituals that enhance the safe passage of the deceased into the next world. Finally, funerals provide an avenue through which the bereaved deal with grief and guilt. Thus, funerals can provide a set of psychologically healthy mourning practices for the bereaved, enabling them to act out their grief in the presence of a support group.

Even though all humans may experience death, conceptions about death and how we respond to issues of death and dying vary widely across cultures. As the world is increasingly shrinking due to the extensive interaction of people from cultures across the world, it is important to understand the complexities that surround the issues of death, just as we do the issues of life. This will better prepare us to respect and understand people from other cultures, and respond to them in ways that are meaningful to them and ourselves so that their lives and ours may be enriched in the process.

MOURNING

In 1982, American psychologist William J. Worden published his book "Grief Counselling and Grief Therapy," which offered his concept of the four tasks of mourning:

Acceptance of the reality of the Loss: Coming to terms with the reality that the person is dead and will not return is the first task. A grieving individual, needs to complete this on their own. The scale of this task depends on the degree of the loss. Example, death of a spouse may cause loss of income, sexual partner, social support, social status, friends etc. Without accomplishing this, one will not be able to continue through the mourning process. This acknowledgement has to be both at the cognitive and emotional levels.

Work Through the Pain of Grief: Reaction to the death of the loved one is often painful, and you will experience a wide range of emotions, such as anger, guilt, fear, depression, sadness, despair, etc. It requires the bereaved to acknowledge these different emotions and the pain, rather than suppressing or avoiding these feelings, in order to work through them. The pain is intense, person might appear to be stuck in guilt, anger, and sadness etc. Trying to avoid pain can actually prolong the course of mourning.

Adjust to an Environment in Which the Deceased is Missing: In addition to emotional adjustments, this task might require adopting a role or function that the deceased once performed, and will vary based on the nature of the relationship. For example, if your spouse or partner dies, this task might involve you handling household finances, raising a child alone etc. This task involves several adjustments – external, internal, a spiritual.

Find a connection with the deceased while embarking on a new life: While nothing can make you to completely forget about your relationship with the deceased, the goal is to find an appropriate place in your emotional life moving forward and to begin living again. This might require letting go of attachments so that new, meaningful relationships can begin to form. The requirements for this fourth task are to find a way for the bereaved to stay connected with the deceased but in ways that enable them embark on their new life without the deceased. This could be by finding a more suitable place for the deceased in the life of the survivor so as to enable the survivor live an effective life.

Working through these four tasks of mourning can help the bereaved come to terms with their loss and return to a new state of normality.

GRIEF HEALING (THE Rs)

There is nothing unemotional about grief and overcoming grief, termed as grief healing. Distress hurts desperately., emotions involved are sharp and unpleasant. Normal life is disrupted, inability to think clearly and sense of loss of meaning in everything necessitates a resolution. An outline and a systematic approach may provide a structure for the process. Some aspects of religious customs already have these aspects inbuilt in them.

Outlined here are linear progressive steps towards managing bereavement process.

a. Recognise: Overcome denial. Release emotions, talk about the loss. Recognise that it is normal to feel depression, regression, anxiety, guilt and withdrawal. You may feel angry, and unreasonable in demands and expectation.
b. Reaffirm: There is no role for guilt, anger, anxiety in the longer-term grieving process. Reaffirm yourself. Start establishing communication with the world outside. Acceptance of reality of loss. Start thinking about other people and their needs. Engaging in funeral and customary activities will help you to reconnect with the world you retreated from.
c. Remove: You have to achieve breaking ties with the diseased person. This may include emotional dependence, loss of sexual partnership, physical dependence on day today activities like cleaning. This does not mean you forget the individual. You start making tasks of adjustment, take vocational responsibility and engage in work activities. You may have to remove certain items to make room in your life.
d. Remember: Promote internal remembrance of the person. If the memories live within you, no one can take it away. This may involve some removal of external items as process of readjustment.
e. Renewal: Loss of a person will require reorganisation of relationship with other friends and family. This may include deepening relationships with other members of family and engaging more time with activities you would have done with the diseased person. Or it may be engaging less with some activities which were primarily related via the diseased person. Change is a good motivation for grief healing.

f. Rediscover: you have to rediscover life and its meaning. Don't be hard on yourself, nothing and no one is permanent including yourself. Life is a journey. Goal is to enjoy the journey, not arriving at a destination because there is none. You arrive at an end.

g. Release: You had a relationship with the person died. Every relationship father to son, husband to wife, or between friend, makes you to commit to certain rules of relationship, some obligations and voluntary restrictions in the code of behaviour. Loss of the relationship will free you from those obligations. You have to appreciate this release. You may not have to do things you did, or you may wish to do somethings differently which you did not consider before. As this could be the precursor to bring about necessary changes to the lifestyle and will help you to cope with the loss.

h. Replacement: no one could be replaced, and dearer the person, larger will be the scale of the loss. However, it is necessary to replace psychological, functional and other social roles you enjoyed with the person you lost. Dying is not the only act when you may lose a person. Similar events may occur during a divorce, child moving out or social distancing. Replacement may not be like for like, could be subliminal or by an object, or totally imaginary.

IMMIGRANTS FACING BEREAVEMENT

Today, more people than ever live in a country other than the one in which they were born. In 2019, the number of migrants globally reached an estimated 272 million, 51 million more than in 2010. International migrants comprise 3.5 per cent of the global population.

When death occurs to a relative in the host country, the bereavement process slightly difficult and complicated by many factors. It is impossible to practice certain significant cultural and religious rituals in the home country. These ritual differences may include timing of the funeral, ways of disposing the physical remains, absence of certain religious input or access to place of worship. Inability to perform these rituals may cause sense of failure and make mourning process difficult.

Immigrants already suffer from multiple loss and bereavement scenarios. These include change in environment, cultural framework, loss of family ties and social status. Additional loss of a person may cause longer term mourning process. Again, most immigrants are not supported in their host country by their family.

Funeral rituals have evolved in response to the rupture in the social fabric caused by death, and the perceived threat from it. Main purpose of such rituals is to prepare the dead for the next life, as believed by the respective religion. But they also give a prescribed structure to the mourning process. The immigrant community either forced to renounce the rituals or adapt the practices of the host society. Most have a hybridized cultural practice to obey the legal structure and framework of the host country and to perform some religious and cultural practices where practical.

WHEN SOMEONE DIES

There are many information resources, to help everyone when they are faced with death of a relative. They cover from documentation to funeral services. Many of us only discover the practical procedures that are necessary after someone dies, when we need to carry them out for a person, we ourselves have loved and are grieving for. Information on where these procedures differ in every country. In many countries, the religious institutes have working arrangement with funeral organisers and will be of immense help. Donation of organs, tissues or the whole body: If the person who is dying or who has died, expressed a wish to donate their organs, their tissues or their whole body, it is essential to inform any professional, involved in their care as soon as possible.

The medical certificate and investigation of the death can be difficult issue, especially if the cremation need to be organised in a short period. After someone dies, their death is usually confirmed by a qualified professional. In a hospital their body will be moved to a mortuary. If a death at home or in a care home had been expected, the body can be moved. If the death was not expected or was not from a natural cause, the person who has died will be moved to a hospital or public mortuary on the instructions of the coroner.

When a death is from known and natural causes, the doctor who has been looking after the person will issue a Medical Certificate of Cause of Death. Hospital staff will explain their arrangements for this if the person died in hospital. If the cause of death is unknown or is not natural, the coroner will investigate the death. This usually requires a post-mortem examination. You will be informed about this by the coroner's office, who will also give you the results. If the death is found to be from a natural cause you will be told how to make an appointment to register the death.

There are some legal and formal documentation and government agency documentation need to be done without delay. Passport Office or identity documents including driving licenses should be returned to the government offices. Tax authorities and banks should be informed of the deceased person. Work place, pensions agency, local council etc. should be informed. It is likely that your household income changed or possibly even dropped when your partner died. But there are things that you can do to make sure that you can take over the finances and keep paying the bills and living within a changed budget. Banks should be informed regarding joint accounts, credit cards and other loans and mortgage accounts. Any formal debt needs to be assigned and included in the estate plan. Insurance cover re car home and life should be updated.

SUMMARY

Grief and loss are universal, no one escapes. Systematic approach to overcome sense of loss is needed. There is less attention in normalising grief process and to help bereaving person to overcome grief. Lot of our efforts are focused on treating abnormal grief and psychotherapy. I have outlined a linear progressive steps one can adapt to overcome grief, what is termed as grief healing.

Pinnacle of Life

KNOW HOW

I see a pheasant, on the road side,

In peace, tranquil, don't know when it died.

Wonder if pheasants have "day of judgement?"

If eaten by a fox, will he pass the test of torment.

No siren, no oxygen, no figures to remember,

No headstone or even a grave to mark its number,

It died at dawn, embraced by a car,

Like an innocent convict hanged to the bar.

Life comes to an end in untold ways,

Plague corona or coronary, only some names.

Be aware, be prepared and stave it off for now,

Live a life, on your terms, I will tell you how.

11 SOLVING THE FINAL MYSTERY.

FINAL MYSTERY

Science has cracked many mysterious aspects of universe, providing us with more and more facts. From prions to boson, from gene therapy to mars landing, science has made leaps which for generations were not even described in fictions. In doing so, science is becoming a subject of the specialist. Even trained scientist can only understand the facts of the top slice of his own field, and rest of it he is as ignorant as any other. Perspective is lost. In doing so we have also lost the ability to comprehend aspects of human life which is not based on facts. The space occupied by theology for long time is getting empty and is not being replaced by anything meaningful. It is quite right that science has expelled mythical beliefs from dictating human life. But it has convincingly failed to provide replacement. There is a mystery to be solved in this aspect of life. More analysis, thinking and perspective and not knowledge and facts is needed in this regard. Death is one such mystery, perhaps the final one we are going to solve. In this chapter and in the epilogue, I will list some ways we can regain that lost perspective.

There is much talk about science doubling our lifespan over last century and perhaps an extrapolation that some further extension could be achieved by generation. Don't get your hopes up, science, as I have already discussed, only partly prevented premature death. Average life span increase is due to smaller proportion of us dying too early. There are more reasons to be prepared.

Look back, focus on yourself.

When you measure remaining life span in decades, you feel no urgency to live your life. Your priorities are to enlarge the horizons of your knowledge, wealth and success to infinity. You wish to make friends, travel to far places, and believe you will go on forever. Looking back, makes you aware how much of your life activity is focused on other people and activities primarily not concerning you. It is time to get some focus on yourself. I do not mean to put yourself under the spotlight for others to see, you may be already doing that. What you need is a focus of introspection, ability to look inside yourself. Consider your fitness, mental health, are you enjoying your job, do you have to do what you are doing or will it be more fulfilling to do something else instead? You do not get younger with time, that is by no means meant to be depressing. It is to put a sense of urgency. Focusing on yourself allows you to hand over some responsibilities and make some room. Good life needs a succession planning.

Look back and start giving

Knowing life is finite, people should give up the destructive greed to amass wealth. Life should be about caring for others, because you like to rather than to collect your pass to go to heaven. Live to grow your knowledge and wisdom, not wealth. You should start to give back. Everyone has something to give, it is matter of attitude. Looking back has advantage of giving you an insight into what you did not do well, what you missed out and what you messed up. Nobody is perfect. But the wise, look back and learn, in time. You do not want to leave it till it is too late. "Dharma" means both duty and giving. Giving does not mean donating all your wealth. You can give education, reassurance, shelter and anything the recipient benefits from. There is more pleasure in giving than you think. You can give time to charitable work, or look after grandchildren or even pledge donating your organs. Giving comes in many forms. Hosting people is a form of giving. People take pride and honour in being a good host.

Appreciate your life.

Life is accumulation of moments. It is amazing to be alive. If life is like a book, you are on a page between the cover pages. We have reason to make the best of this world, because we know there is no other. No matter how difficult everyday living may be sometimes, seeing our lives in this wider context can help us to put everyday worries into perspective. In the history of the planet earth your life span is a mere flash of light. And you are in that flash, at this moment. Remind yourself this fact regularly. You are the lucky one.

See life as the exception, not the norm. Too often we focus on life as normal and death as an exception. Some time it is true, but we always know death is inevitable. Life has to be an exception. Feeling lucky is not just because you are alive. Practically you are alive in this technological era of human domination in technology allowing you better access to health travel and leisure. Philosophically you can count lucky to be born as a human on the beautiful planet. We do not need any wealth, wisdom or success to appreciate life, neither you need to be thankful to anyone for it! There is indeed a lot to lose when you die, but if you appreciated all that when you had it, you can be at ease that once you die, this will not matter to you.

Work longer

People need to remain in work for longer, perhaps until they actually can physically do so. Of course, you can reduce amount and complexity of work, and perhaps change the pattern of work to suit your capabilities. Working longer in life has many advantages, to employee, employer and the society or government as a whole. Longer working life actually help to keep your brain function in better shape, and keeps your life style active. Attending your workplace regularly ensures you do not feel lonely and you will feel valued in the society. The cliff edge changes the retirement brings to your life is eventual detrimental to your psychological wellbeing. Further ability to work longer means you earn longer, feel less forced to save up large amount of money towards retirement and be able to spend and have better quality of life. Working till later in life also means you will have shorter old age without earnings, which also means you can afford better quality of care when you really need it, when you become dependent.

Employees should encourage older employees to remain in work by making necessary changes to the work place needs. Older employees are more experienced, loyal, and perhaps need less training and support. Also, they are more likely to be flexible, able to work evenings, summer holidays, weekends by not having fixed family commitments. Longer working life will enable employers to be flexible about the pay structure and reduces burden of pension pay outs. Society and government as a whole will be benefitted by the elderly workforce. They are paying taxes, productive and less likely to strain the public purse by using public services. However, this process needs fundamental changes to the way we look after the elderly. Old people will have higher need to see their doctor, more often for example. An elderly lady in the work force should be able to see her doctor at the choice of her time, and not having to wait for months to make an appointment.

Beware of medical excess

The fear of death is most unjustified of all fears, for there is no risk of accidents for someone who is dead. - Albert Einstein

Doctors including, every medical professional do their very best to keep patients alive, healthy, free of pain and suffering and try to keep you free of disease. But in the process, inadvertently they may affect your wellbeing, because wellbeing is not just about being free of an ailment. In the process of medical intervention, your quality of life may deteriorate so much, that you might have preferred not to have gone through the treatment. Medical treatment sometimes, appear defensive, evasive and medicolegally driven rather than guided by the wants of the patient. The culture needs to change. Our medical system is not relevant to the dying, many doctors have no experience in dealing with the end of life. Medical professionals are emotionally detached from the patients. Beware of the tubes, pipes, bags, cylinders, monitors, humidifiers and other intelligent devices which may surround you on your last days. Would rather not have these, just a kiss of good bye from dear one, a sip of medication to alleviate pain and anxiety, and a warm blanket would perhaps your choice, or even someone sitting to you and reading a holy scripture letting you pass into eternal sleep. Debate needs to happen among the learned people, medical professionals, care institutes. Is that science fit for purpose?

I have a question, and do not know the answer to, I will write about it, hopefully someone will answer it to themselves. A preventive medication, example Statins. Even though controversial, a death preventive strategy. Benefits of statins are realised over decades. Do we need to keep giving them to everyone, even when they turn ninety? What are we trying to prevent? Similar argument then can be expanded to many preventive medicalisation of the elderly. Then in reverse, a nihilistic behaviour, like diet or smoking, again take decades to cause real harm. Will it be safe to say, with progression of age the real harm caused by health related nihilistic behavior is really low? I am not saying we should encourage all elderly to take up smoking. Just our resources and focus of death preventive strategy including medication should focus on where it really matters. Is it health effective or cost effective to keep taking antihypertensives until we die?

Better understanding the dying process can help us stop treating death as a medical problem to be fixed, and instead as an inevitability that should be as comfortable and peaceful as possible. For this you should have the courage to live, even if it means dying a little earlier than the experts, and even our families, might insist.

Life does go on

This is what you would hear if they say something,

"Life should go on, and change nothing."

They have seen it all in their life and dying,

the dead ask nothing from the living.

Almost every single person has deep seated worries about what happens to their near and dear after their death. This arises from self or egocentric view of the world. Person imagines that their future absence from day today role may cause potential or actual harm to their loved one. The better the relationship role the person plays, the stronger is the anxiety and fear. Mothers worry about future of children, husbands about their wife. Owners of pets worry about the future of their beloved pet after their demise. Yes, it is undoubtedly a big change and sometimes a challenge for the bereaved family or pet or even a company or a nation to come to terms with loss of a person. It creates a void, which requires others to fill in the space. Some space will never be filled. But life goes on. Nature and society have dealt with these events for generations. It is not a source of anxiety. Sooner you develop the concept that you are not the center of the social function, allow others to take that role, develop detachment and facilitate the transition, the smoother it will be for the people you leave behind to cope with the loss. The transition can take days or decades depending on the circumstances, make a start. You may not accomplish the order and degree of transfer you wish, but it is better than doing nothing, further, more it is far better than not doing anything and just worrying.

If you are relative of someone nearing end of life, there is something you can do to help them. Just tell them, if they do go, "you will be alright". This will be huge relief to them and help them to focus their energy on themselves rather than worry about you. It is not in form being disrespectful or being indifferent to all the things the person has done for you. It is a way of promoting that detachment, facilitating the release, the true meaning of Nirvana.

Make life worth living

Prohibit the talking of omens, and do away with superstitious doubts. Then until death itself comes, no calamity needs to be feared. – Sun Tzu

Often health care settings, or elderly residences have regimental rules for the residents. The rules reflect the madness of political correctness and safety culture the society largely suffers from. Would you like stop your grandmother drinking her favourite tipple because it is bad for her health? Would you stop a ninety-year-old diabetic uncle from helping himself to a bar of chocolate because his HbA1c may shoot up? Let them live, these are elderly, let them enjoy what is left of their life. Give them pleasure, comfort and care. Not safety and rule books. Care homes should be homes first, were the person has the freedom dignity and privacy, to decide when and what care they need, not dictated by the law of medicines and professionalism of the care home staff. People should retain the ability to decide how to spend their time, space and possessions during their ripe old days. Life is worth living in any condition, even when you are old, frail and can't fend for yourself any longer. There is a purpose for life even when you are looking imminently to the end. End, it is the pinnacle, it is the apex and the ultimate life's experience.

Thinking about death all the time, however, is paralyzing. Forgetting about death is just as important as remembering it. Everything should be in moderation, even reflection. If you spend all your time thinking that you will not be around someday, you could lose motivation to do what you have to do in life. At its extreme, anxiety or fear of death can be a health disorder.

Holding on or Letting Go

"Mostly it is the loss which teaches us about the worth of things" – Arthur Schopenhauer

When we realize that the end of life may be approaching, other thoughts and feelings arise. The person who is ill will want to be with loved ones, visit the place where they grew up. They may also feel a sense of responsibility towards the dependents or relatives and not wanting to fail them nor cause them grief. Even in facing death, hope remains. As a bargaining stage, we may hope for a restful night, or another visit with a particular friend, or just a quiet passing from this life.

The Jewish prayer of the gravely ill puts it well for both the person who is ill and the loved ones caring for him "I do not choose to die. May it come to pass that I may be healed. But if death is my fate, then I accept it with dignity."

And holding on to life, to our loved ones, is indeed a basic human instinct. However, as the end comes closer, due to feeling of loss of control or suffering, person changes the attitude and starts to "let go". As death nears, many people feel a lessening of their desire to live longer. This is different from depression or thoughts of suicide. Instead, they sense it is time to let go. Perhaps, as in other times in life, it's a sense that it's time for a major change like one might feel when moving away from home, getting married, divorcing or changing to a new job. Some people describe a profound tiredness, a tiredness that no longer goes away with rest. Others may reach a point where they feel they have struggled as much as they have been called upon to do and will struggle no more. Refusing to let go can prolong dying, but it cannot prevent it. Dying, thus prolonged, can become more a time of suffering than of living.

Family members and friends who love the dying person may experience a similar change. At first, one may adjust to managing a chronic illness, then learn to accept a life limiting illness, and then accept the possibility of a loved one dying. Some may refuse to accept the inevitability of death. Lastly, one may see that dying is the better of two choices, and be ready to give the loved one permission to die. As mentioned, the dying may be distressed at causing grief for those who love them, and, receiving permission to die can relieve their distress.

When you are gone, you are gone.

For death and life are one, even as the river and sea are one – Poetry, Kahlil Gibran

When I die, I die and I am gone. My consciousness and interaction with everything and everyone are gone. My afterlife only remains with those who carry my memories. "You're not really dead until everyone who knew you is dead too." The sense that life is finite, now and here is a beautiful concept. No heaven, no hell, no judgement, no cycles, and no awaiting rewards. It is all now and here for me to live, every moment of it.

Planning for your own death, whether that is expected or not, takes a lot of time and energy to complete. It is much better to take the time now, while you have it, to lay out your plans, wishes, directions and desires, so your passing will be peaceful, for both you, your family and friends. We start ageing from the day we are born, and the clock starts ticking.

Reject superstitious beliefs

There is a very popular opinion that choosing life is inherently superior to choosing death. This belief that life is inherently preferable to death is one of the most widespread superstitions, the bias constitutes on of the most obstinate mythologies of the human species. – Author Mitchell Heisman.

Modern society does not want to see death, in any form. We don't have time to wait for it, even when it occurs in most docile way. We expect death to be performed out of sight, presented cleaned and attractively packaged, ready for us to lay the flowers of tribute, at our time of convenience. We are comfortable to pay tribute to the dead but not associate with the death or dying process. Well, is that all you care about the person dying? The main reason for disassociation of death from normal society is superstitious beliefs. Also, biologically we view death as unglamorous act perhaps, like outcast untouchable. As humans we all have inconvenience from certain things we do, like we burp, fart, vomit, sneeze, dribble, menstruate etc. We have acceptance of these. Yes, death is not pretty, sometimes can be associated with unpleasant sight. But it is physiologic activity, perhaps the last of the dying person. There is a need to be real and not superstitious about death.

When death occurs, many cultures the grieving wear symbolic colours to depict something bad has happened, follow activities like not wearing jewellery, not listen to music or not eating certain food. In some communities, family remain isolated for a short period. Some of these customs help the bereaved family but they should be an option and compulsion.

Accepting death

"To begin depriving death of its greatest advantage over us, let us adopt a way clean contrary to that common one; let us deprive death of its strangeness, let us frequent it, let us get used to it; let us have nothing more often in mind than death. We do not know where death awaits us, so let us wait for it everywhere. To practice death is to practice freedom. A man who has learned how to die has unlearned how to be a slave."
Michel de Montaigne.

Comforting thing about our own death is that there is nothing we can do about it when it happens.

So, although it may be intensely sad to leave behind all the things that come with being an experiencing creature, if we can come to terms with the fact that we have no choice but to leave them behind, we can allow ourselves a more peaceful, fulfilling death. For some people this acceptance doesn't happen until near the very end of life, but it is part of letting go.

This is of course simply a general comment about the moment of death. And it doesn't mean that we don't have choice and control in our end of life care depending on how our life is ending – indeed, this sense of empowerment can be vital to our ability to have a 'good death'.

Knowing about your death

Death is a word, it is the word, the image that creates fear –
Jiddu Krishnamurthy.

None of us really know what death truly is like. But in order to have realistic prospective and expectation, we need to understand the process as best as possible. Having unmet expectations make the process of death difficult for the dying and the families. Specially, medical interventions made at near end of life can be of questionable benefit. By understanding the reality of the process, we and our bodies may well go through when we die, we may well gain the final inspiration. Death, when it comes, doesn't often take place in a way that we would see as dignified while we are healthy.

For many, thinking about death, or even reading this book is not comfortable and daunting. When you are engaged in the reality of normal day to day life, you start to feel it is extreme to think about your own death. This is because it is an extreme, potentially life changing knowledge and realisation about our life's reality. Also, very few people around you have spent any time to try and understand, or not have accepted the facts of life. Coming to terms with one's death involves reflection on its significance in one's life, and thinking about the larger values that give life its meaning.

Q : Once you acknowledge death, can you still lead a normal life?

Of many issues I discuss with younger generation, this question often bothers them when they start looking at death awareness. I felt I should address this in the book. I think many of you are concerned that once start contemplating death, dying and issues around end of life, you will become detached from real material life, become reclusive and start living in hermitage.

Not true, acknowledgement, awareness and preparedness of death will certainly allow you to live a life more meaningful than otherwise. Live every day like today is your last day on planet, you will value everything and enjoy everyone a little more. You will get a bit more out of your time. This does not preclude you from long term planning, work harder, motivate yourself to acquire knowledge, wealth and wisdom. You will have better perspective of life. Better balance. Perhaps you will not work that harder, chase mirage of wealth, do anything unethical to amass wealth. working harder today to gather wealth with a view of better life tomorrow is not always a good attitude. If you only focus on gathering wealth, and do not enjoy your life, or feel that you do not have time, yes, tomorrow will definitely a better be a better life, but just it may not be your life. Remember, once you are gone, you are gone. You take nothing from here.

Hermitage of life in Sannyasa will reduce bondage with materialistic life as I discussed in the bucket list. However, with death awareness you do not have to live like recluse, you can have all the pleasure of the material world along with realism of life and death.

I have discussed about immortality and how it is not possible to achieve it in a meaningful way. Having established that, you will probably focus better of needs of other people than egocentric self. That is act of true humanity. And I hope by the time you come to end of life, your account with this planet and its resources will be in good balance.

Q : "Thinking about death" Isn't it distracting and disturbing?

Yes, it can be. Most thoughts, conflicts and facts about death are subconscious in our mind. Anything involving subconscious mind provoke strong emotional and primitive thoughts. This can disturb a predominantly frontal cortex based, day to day life. This is true in any event when you provoke such response. This may include watching a disturbing film, reading a book of horror or any other social events. In the subconscious, there are fears, fear of unknown, fear of loss, fear of pain and death encompasses all those fears and many more. Therefore, thinking about death can bring about distraction from normal thinking.

Can we afford not to think about it? Absolutely not. Not thinking about anything disturbing is societies response, and is not effective way of dealing with a problem. People seem to keep themselves preoccupied in the modern era, may it be productive work or media entertainment, allowing themselves to shut away from thinking about any issues which are disturbing. Thinking about death all the time and preoccupied by it is pathological. But the approach should be to bring the issue to the frontal cortex. Not to view it as a fearful event, try and understand it, I called it a business like, approach. Make specific decisions and act on awareness, preparedness and not ponder on it all the time.

SUMMARY - **Live happy to die happy.**

I am not trying to tell you how to live happy, you already know that. But further emphasis, it is important to live happy, to be able to die happy.

Make a "bucket list" of things you want to do, places you want to go, experiences you want to have in the time you have left. It may not be all fun, there may be issues you would like to reconcile, people you wish to apologise, share your feelings. Get them out of the way. Work at checking things off the list. Enjoy yourself along the way. Realize that having a "bucket list" and working to get items checked off, provides a subtle reminder that one day, maybe sooner, maybe later, yours will be kicked.

Pinnacle of Life

WISDOM

Your heart was beating before you were born
And your legacy remains after you are gone.
Before the beginning and after the end,
where the time immortal and infinite blend,

If life is an illusion, then you have done well
to remain visible in the short spell,
Life goes beyond realms of birth and death
Enjoy it to the fullest while you still have your breath,

There is a trade-off between nature and mankind,
Nature of the nature, to mop up, leave nothing behind,
Be aware, be prepared and make a good deal and carry on,
Life is at your feet, celebrate, cherish and enjoy, my son.

Epilogue: Pillars of Wisdom.

Death is often described as the end result and loss in a struggle. Perhaps sometime we can describe it, as end result and a victory in a struggle. After all, "The surprise is not that we die, but that we live, for so long and successfully, in the face of all the morbid risks of life". We are not cursed, but blessed to die, just we do not appreciate the fact. Death remains a mystery. Leave it to medicine, science, philosophy and politicians to deal with the enigma.

There are some things you can do to have sense of control towards end of your life. I have called them the **pillars of wisdom.**

- Become death aware.
- Be death prepared.
- Adopt death preventive behaviour.
- Live fulfilling life.
- Decide your own pathway.

Adopting the five pillars of thoughts will help you to achieve sense of control, ease you on the path of unknown destiny. It will help others to deal with your demise and allows them to celebrate your life. It reduces strain and anxiety on you and your loved one. Make a simple start, this is not science, philosophy, cult or religion. There are no formulas or scriptures. Take small steps. Every little step takes you to that far closer.

Become **death aware** is about thinking and talking about your own death.

- Volunteer at a hospice.
- Read a book about bereavement.
- Think for a moment where you would like to die, ideally.
- Talk to your friend about what you would like at your funeral.
- Talk to your family about your legacy.
- Write Your Own Obituary.

Being **death prepared** is to acknowledge loss, mitigate risk, detachment and reflection.

- Take a life insurance policy.
- Write a will.
- Do some decluttering of personal belongings.
- Go on a holiday away from your family, make some space.
- Handover some responsibilities and authority to younger generation.
- Create an income stream by investing carefully.

Death preventive behaviour is best way of how not to welcome death. Eat only what you have to, adopt active physical and social life, preventive medical intervention etc. You know what is best for you.

- Have a medical check-up.
- Take regular walks.
- Go vegetarian for a month.
- Moderate alcohol intake.
- Take up yoga and relaxation.

Live fulfilling life, don't look for meaning of your life, resist micromanagement, ignore superstitions and be mindful. Do good.

- Plant a tree.
- Work for a charity.
- Teach your skills to others.
- Donate part of your wealth.
- Communicate with an old friend, write a letter.

Decide **your own pathway**. First what is that you don't want and then, where possible what is that you want.

- Your decision about legacy pathways.
- Your views about CPR, blood transfusion, use of sedatives at end of life.
- Your views about hospice care, home death, presence of family.
- Your wishes about disposal of physical remains.
- Your views about celebrating your life after you are gone.
- Appoint a power of attorney for health issues

When you have done a bit of the all five steps then go back and do again a bit more, and then again.

WHY THESE PILLARS

Scene of death has been pushed out of our sight and we panic when we come to face it. Thought of death has been driven deep into our unconscious. From there the paradoxical thought of reality versus denial keep troubling our mind. The strain caused by the conflict might result in personality disorders and somatic illness like hypertension. We need to bring the sight and thought of death to conscious mind and make it visible. Hence the first pillar "Death awareness". Objective of death awareness is to make death less strange. It is not a new concept, in fact there is explosion of death awareness literature, training and concepts in recent years. Both Freud and Becker, may be right or wrong in their conflicting theories about death and the unconscious. Important issue is how to resolve the conflict. Release of this subliminal thought will result in better acceptance, better knowledge and therefore better social attitude towards death. Certainly, this will help in reducing death anxiety.

Twentieth century witnessed expression of sex, sexuality and sexual attitude brought into conscious mind. The resultant expression of freedom, removal of taboo and social acceptance has led to revolutionary changes in our society. A similar change and acceptance about death, way we die and what control we can have on it, is needed. Education is the key. Death awareness is the pillar to support that change.

Very similar to how the thought of death has been pushed back into our subconscious, the timing of our death has been pushed out of our sight. Modern life has made us think death is far away somewhere and we don't need to prepare for it. When, in circumstances, death occurs suddenly or with short notice, we can't believe it, we try to deny this till the inevitable. The major shock during COVID was not just the numbers, but it is the fact that death occurred in people which was unacceptable or outside the norms we got used to. But it is the character of death, it is the most predictable and most unpredictable event. "Death preparedness" is the pillar of building an acceptance approach to this unpredictability. There is no ideal time when you wish to start. First time, you pause, look back at your own life and decided what you are getting right and what you like to change, that is the moment you have already started death preparedness. It is not welcoming death or enjoying it's coming. It is getting your baton ready to handover in the relay. It is mitigating risks to others in case of your loss.

Accepting and acknowledging the mortality, should help you reduce your attachment to the materialistic world. Hope is that it should reduce the need to rely on the rat race and stop you from excesses of wealth. The nature of wealth is such, you are always unhappy at any amount of wealth you have or you don't have. And there is static amount, by definition if one has too much, many will have too little. If we all have to live well, we all need comfort and happiness, not too much work, success, wealth and fame. Death is a great equaliser; the knowledge should enhance universal brotherhood (Vishwa bhrata concept from Vivekananda).

Third pillar for the individual and the society is the "death prevention". Having understood the concept of unpredictable but inevitable nature of death, we need to defer death as best as possible, until desired. Prevention of death is like any other preventive program. In COVID individual level preventive strategy involved washing hands, social distancing measures, working from home where possible and reduce contact with high risk groups. Primary prevention at community and nation level included lock down, prevention of cross border travel and cancellation of flights. In a way everything we do day to day is death prevention!

Global level, we can do more, vaccination, clean drinking water, promoting hygiene and sanitation, prevention of nutritional deficiencies and infections. We had some success in reducing smoking, but rising incidence of diabetes, level of alcohol consumption and obesity are threatening increasing mortality in younger population. Individual level, everyone can design their own preventive program. First identify the specific risk and then try to reduce the risk exposure. Reduction in nihilistic attitude, abiding by the health and safety advice and life style changes are all part of preventive behaviour.

Living a full life in all dimensions and be satisfied with it is probably the best preparation for dying. Hence the pillar of "fulfilled life". There is no meaning in life, do not waste your time, but rather think about giving meaning to life, your own life, on your own. You know what you want to do from what you have got. Make the most of it. Have a bucket list and go for it. Reality will preclude you from some things you wish to do, but you should know your limits. Sometime don't look at the mirror, look in your mind, mind reflects better than mirror. The objective is not to have regrets, guilt or unfulfilled desires, when you have to decide the day has come. One small note, having the latest model of gadget is not necessarily fulfilment of your life, it is short term materialistic vision. Because before end of your time, or in a year's time you will need to keep up with the next model!

Last and perhaps most difficult to achieve, the pillar is "Deciding your own pathway". This is real preparation to your departure, and will involve dialogue with other people, their support and agreement to achieve. Other characteristic of this pillar is, it is primarily to benefit of others as well as to ease your way to exit. Animal welfare standards dictate reducing anxiety in cattle before they are taken to slaughterhouse. Deciding your own pathway is same. Every possible action you can take to, to be sure, decisive and guide other what they should and should not do in case of your incapacity or death, help them to help your better. There is no better legacy to leave to your children than a well-planned exist, decluttered and defined.

There are barriers to achieve these goals. You have to systematically approach these, by making very small changes and steps. It is tempting to attend an intensive course on dying and be fully prepared. But it is not the knowledge and lectures you need. The dire need is reflection and acceptance. That can only happen gradually. We can also think of introducing death education in curriculum same as relationship education. Again, it is probably age appropriate for older population who look back, and live in the past to have reflection. Attitude of family members could be a difficult barrier to overcome. Your family members find it unacceptable for you to start thinking about death. Well, the detachment has to start some time, acceptance has to happen, longer the time you have to make everyone aware of your wishes, the easier it will be in the end. Life style, financial commitments and obligations could prevent you from discussing issues of your death. You only need to make a small start.

It is not easy to detach from this world's maya.

Pinnacle of Life

INSPIRATION

I am immensely grateful to many authors and publications whose material inspired me to write. I have borrowed generously from the richness of the ideas. I have made a small list, useful for further exploration.

- Aries, Philippe (1981): *The Hour of our Death*, translated by Helen Weaver.
- Becker, Earnest (1973) *The Denial of Death*.
- Cave, Stephen (2012) *Immortality, The quest to live forever and how it drives civilization*.
- Durant, Will (1926) *The Story of Philosophy*.
- Dawkins, Richard (1976) *The selfish gene*.
- Gaskin, John (translation) (1995) *The Epicurean Philosophers*.
- Gawande, Atul (2014) *Being Mortal: Illness, Medicine and What Matters in the End*.
- Kalanithi, Paul (2017) *When breath becomes air*.
- Kubler-Ross, Elisabeth (1969) *On Death and Dying*.
- Michael Hebb and Angela Grant (2016) *Let's talk about Death over Dinner*
- Nuland, Sherwin B. (1994) *How we die*.
- O'Mahony Seamus (2016) *The way we die now*.
- Switzer, David (1970) *The Dynamics of grief*.
- Tolstoy, L. 2006 (1886). *The Death of Ivan Ilyich*.
- Walter Tony (1994) *The Revival of Death*. Routledge
- Zackhiem, Victoria, (2012) *Exit Laughing : How humour takes the sting out of death*.
- www.lifesquared.org.uk : *How to think about death (and life)* pdf leaflet.
- www.dyingmatters.org : *Understanding death and dying*.

Pinnacle of Life

ABOUT THE AUTHOR

"Pinnacle of life" is the first literary work from KISHORE SHANBHAG. He is an Associate specialist in the department of Oral and Maxillofacial Surgery, East Lancashire Hospitals NHS Trust, Blackburn. He was born in India and completed his graduation and master's degree in Dentistry from SDM College of Dental Sciences Dharwad, India. Following his fellowship examination from Royal College of Surgeons of Edinburgh, he joined the National Health Service, United Kingdom and served in various positions. His writing is influenced by his upbringing in rural Indian setting, life in the United Kingdom, his medical experience and love of reading books. He lives in Bolton, UK with his wife Kanchan and daughter Tejal.

Pinnacle of Life

www.ingramcontent.com/pod-product-compliance
Lightning Source LLC
Chambersburg PA
CBHW071356210526
45465CB00001B/116